The Anthropology of Child and Youth Care Work

The Anthropology of Child and Youth Care Work

Rivka A. Eisikovits

Jerome Beker
Journal Editor

Child & Youth Services
Volume 18, Number 1

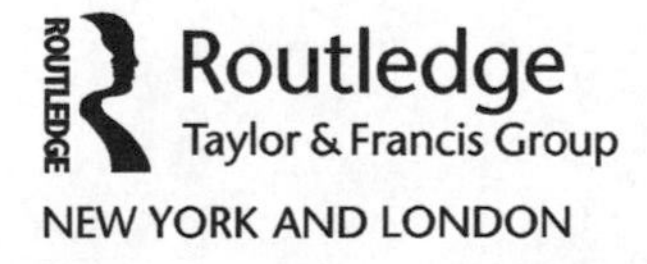

NEW YORK AND LONDON

The Anthrpology of Child and Youth Care Work has also been published as *Child & Youth Services,* Volume 18, Number 1 1997.

First published 1997 by

The Haworth Press, Inc., 10 Alice Street, Binghamton, NY 13904-1580 USA

This edition published 2012 by Routledge

Routledge
Taylor & Francis Group
711 Third Avenue
New York, NY 10017, USA

Routledge
Taylor & Francis Group
2 Park Square Milton Park,
Abingdon Oxfordshire OX14 4RN

First issued in paperback 2016

Routledge is an imprint of the Taylor and Francis Group, an informa business

Library of Congress Cataloging-In-Publication Data

Eisikovits, Rivka Anne.
The anthropology of child and youth care work / Rivka A. Eisikovits.
p. cm.
"Has also been published as Child & youth services, volume 18 number I. I997"-T.p. verso.
Includes bibliographical references (p.) and index.
ISBN 1-56024-848-3 (alk. paper)
1. Social work with children-Research -Methodology. 2. Social work with youth-Research-Methodology. I. Title
HV7I3. E47 1997 96-33326
362.7-dc20 CIP

ISBN 13: 978-1-138-98877-4 (pbk)
ISBN 13: 978-1-56024-848-4 (hbk)

ABOUT THE AUTHOR

Rivka A. Eisikovits, PhD, is Associate Professor of Anthropology and Education at the University of Haifa, Israel, where she is also Chair of The Educational Foundations Program and Head of the Laboratory for the Study of Cultural and Cross-Cultural Learning. Dr. Eisikovits is co-editor of *Qualitative Research and Evaluation in Group Care* and co-author of *Culture Acquisition: A Holistic Approach to Human Learning* (1989). Her publications on the anthropology of group care settings, professional learning, the cross-cultural adaptation of immigrant students, and the philosophy of research methodology have appeared in U.S., European, and Israeli journals.

The Anthropology of Child and Youth Care Work

Child & Youth Services
Volume 18, Number 1

CONTENTS

Foreword

In common with other professional specializations within the broad field of human services, work with children and youth is viewed by most of us who are involved in it as a multidisciplinary field that draws on (and contributes to) the expertise of a variety of academic and professional sources in building its base of knowledge and practice. In this connection, we have long been "teased" by anthropology, sensing that it is a discipline with much to teach us, although we have usually been unable to access its potential in a systematic way. There have been a variety of contributions to our literature by anthropologists and others writing from an anthropological perspective, prominently including the work of Rivka Eisikovits, but its usefulness has mostly been limited to specific applications.

With the publication of this book, things have changed. Not only has Eisikovits presented an overview of how anthropological knowledge and method can advance the field, which she has done elsewhere before, but she has grounded that explicitly in the examples provided by her specific studies and detailed their relevance for practice and their implications for knowledge development and the further enhancement of practice in the future. Although set in the context of residential group care, treatment, and education programs, the information and approach have implications for work with young people in other settings and, indeed, for work with people of all ages. Readers who are familiar with the kinds of settings to which she refers will recognize them, and perhaps themselves, in her words and those of the participants whom she quotes.

[Haworth co-indexing entry note]: "Foreword." Beker, Jerome. Co-published simultaneously in *Child & Youth Services* (The Haworth Press, Inc.) Vol. 18, No. 1, 1997, pp. xv-xvi; and: *The Anthropology of Child and Youth Care Work* (Rivka A. Eisikovits) The Haworth Press, Inc., 1997, pp. xv-xvi. Single or multiple copies of this article are available from The Haworth Document Delivery Service [1-800-342-9678, 9:00 a.m. - 5:00 p.m. (EST). E-mail address: getinfo@haworth.com].

The book can be used on several levels: to illuminate effective practice for direct service workers, to provide the basis for more effective pre- and in-service training, to assess and enhance organizational functioning, and to guide knowledge development to advance all of these purposes in the future. In these ways, it should enable the field to enlist the insights of anthropology as it has those of other behavioral and social sciences in the service of children and youth.

It turns out, I think many readers will agree, that the anthropological perspective has at least as much to contribute as have others that have been applied to the field over the years, and Eisikovits has drawn on her extensive experiential knowledge of child and youth care settings as well as her considerable academic expertise to produce this book. Those who have read her work before–and it appears frequently throughout the relevant literature–will recall that she is also a careful and precise writer who blends these two fields clearly and productively. We will be better practitioners, supervisors, teachers, and researchers for having read this book.

Jerome Beker
Editor
Child & Youth Services
University of Minnesota

Acknowledgments

First of all I wish to thank Jerome Beker for his sustained interest in my work and for his encouragement in putting this volume together. I am also grateful to Wayne Fox, Director of the Center for Developmental Disabilities at the University of Vermont, for his friendship and personal support, to the Center for institutional assistance, and to the University of Haifa for a full academic year sabbatical leave. I would like to acknowledge Gail Manzi, who typed the manuscript, for her professional work and patience. My deepest gratitude is due to my husband, Zvi, for being my lifelong friend and colleague. From his unwavering confidence in me I derived the energy to complete this project. Finally, special thanks to my son, Nir, for being a constant source of joy and inspiration in my life.

Introduction

This book reflects my evolving relationship with the field of child and youth care work over a period of a decade and a half. It started out as a research involvement, i.e., an educational anthropologist doing fieldwork in a residential setting for delinquent girls from which a number of cultural studies of this intriguing world resulted (Eisikovits, 1980, 1983; Eisikovits & Eisikovits, 1980).

My child and youth care worker informants, who gradually became active research partners (Spradley, 1980), discovered the usefulness of this perspective for making better sense of their work. To facilitate the systematic application of the approach in these contexts I reconceptualized the fieldwork experience as a cohesive working model which I called the Child Care Worker as an Ethnographer (Eisikovits, 1991). In the course of experimenting with it, however, I realized that the "ethnographer" label, which mainly refers to anthropological fieldwork including its methodological aspects (Wolcott, 1994), does not encapsulate all the dimensions of this interprofessional analogy. The conceptual frameworks the model provides to assist in analyzing and interpreting the collected data–such as cultural learning, culture change, and systems theories, to name only a few–are not covered. Therefore the approach is referred to as "anthropological" or "cultural" throughout the book, except when issues directly related to fieldwork are addressed.

Wolcott (1982) makes a distinction between the use of ethnographies as "mirrors" or as "models" by various audiences. Some of the texts that appear in this volume were originally written as "mirrors," but in their present form several are transformed into "mod-

---

[Haworth co-indexing entry note]: "Introduction." Eisikovits, Rivka A. Co-published simultaneously in *Child & Youth Services* (The Haworth Press, Inc.) Vol. 18, No. 1, 1997, pp. 1-3; and: *The Anthropology of Child and Youth Care Work* (Rivka A. Eisikovits) The Haworth Press, Inc., 1997, pp. 1-3. Single or multiple copies of this article are available from The Haworth Document Delivery Service [1-800-342-9678, 9:00 a.m. - 5:00 p.m. (EST). E-mail address: getinfo@haworth.com].

els." While Wolcott refers to models for *writing* ethnography, these are models for *doing* ethnography. A preface to each chapter addresses the intricacies of this epistemological metamorphosis.

Various ethnographic styles prevail in anthropology, ranging from emphasis on systematic data collection and description (Dobbert & Kurth-Shai, 1992; LeCompte & Preissle with Tesch, 1993; Pelto & Pelto, 1978; Werner & Schoepfle, 1981a,b; Wolcott, 1994), through concern with interpretation (Frankel, 1987; Geertz, 1973, 1988; Sanjek, 1990, 1991), to the post-modernist preoccupation with the interrelationship between the ethnographer and those being studied, as reflected in both the fieldwork process and its outcomes (Atkinson, 1992; Clifford, 1986; Paget, 1990; Rose, 1990).

The selections included here range in style from descriptive, to interpretive or comparative. Others are critical or programmatic, as a function of the message they have to convey. Fieldwork, as used in this book, is both an experience and a state of mind. The image of the classical anthropologist striving to unravel the mysteries of a foreign culture is offered as a source of inspiration, indeed, a role model for child and youth care workers. Learning to render the familiar strange and then familiar again (Spindler, 1982) in order to see it in a new light is an empowering prospect for people so intensely engaged in the lives of those they work with.

Chapter 1 explains the model and presents the theoretical approach of anthropology and the ethnographic style of inquiry, contextualized in child and youth care worker education and practice settings. It is broadly conceptualized to serve as a basis for application by educators in the field, organizers of in-service training programs, administrators, supervisory and consultative personnel who wish to adopt this perspective for education, training, or practice, in residential as well as non-residential service delivery contexts.

Chapter 2 illustrates the uses of ethnographic description for professional education. Chapter 3 undertakes a critical analysis of staff-client relations, based on fieldwork conducted in a residential setting for girls. Practice implications are highlighted. Studying the interaction styles between organizational subsystems in two child and youth care settings comparatively, Chapter 4 looks at their educational outcomes as experienced by clients.

Chapter 5 combines a cultural and heuristic futures perspective to explore the potential of the residential education alternative for a variety of youthful populations. An instrument for cultural sensitization of practitioners called "Family Culture Ethnography" is presented in Chapter 6. It is brought here as one illustration of the anthropological model's operational potential. Some concluding remarks examine the promise of this approach for the field of child and youth care work.

Chapter 1

An Anthropological Model for Child and Youth Care Worker Education and Practice

While I was doing anthropological fieldwork in a residential treatment center for delinquent and emotionally challenged adolescent girls, a unique relationship developed between myself and child and youth care workers in the setting. To better understand the culture of this institution I worked as a part-time youth counselor (local term for direct care worker) and communication consultant for the 18-month duration of the study. All participants, workers as well as clients, were aware of this research activity. The following excerpt from Eisikovits (1980, p. 159) is illustrative:

> During the weekly team meetings, I would take a few minutes to read some of my field notes to the team members for correction and feedback. Here are some typical reactions:
>
> "Is this really what we sound like?"
> "Could all this make sense to an outsider?"

This is a substantially revised and enlarged version of R. A. Eisikovits, "The Child Care Worker as Ethnographer: Uses of the Anthropological Approach in Residential Child and Youth Care Worker Education and Practice." In J. Beker & Z. Eisikovits (Eds.), *Knowledge Utilization in Residential Child and Youth Care Practice*. Child Welfare League of America, 1991. It is used here with the permission of the editors and the publisher.

[Haworth co-indexing entry note]: "An Anthropological Model for Child and Youth Care Worker Education and Practice." Eisikovits, Rivka A. Co-published simultaneously in *Child & Youth Services* (The Haworth Press, Inc.) Vol. 18, No. 1, 1997, pp. 5-20; and: *The Anthropology of Child and Youth Care Work* (Rivka A. Eisikovits) The Haworth Press, Inc., 1997, pp. 5-20. Single or multiple copies of this article are available from The Haworth Document Delivery Service [1-800-342-9678, 9:00 a.m. - 5:00 p.m. (EST). E-mail address: getinfo@haworth.com].

> "Isn't that ridiculous how much time we spent on her?"
> "He was speaking all the time, making all the decisions."
>
> Gradually they started using my field notes to evaluate their group process. These both stimulated them and provided that minimal distance necessary to contemplate their own actions.

This practice helped to reduce suspicion and to dissociate my note-taking from such activities as periodic peer reviews, which also took place during these meetings. The latter involved tape recording of sessions and had direct bearing on participants' career advancement.

In spite of the incidental nature of their exposure to the anthropological perspective, these child and youth care workers came to recognize–or, rather, to intuit–its practice-enhancing potential. This, in turn, prompted a more thorough investigation of the rapprochement on my part, to try to explain why the anthropological "lenses" fit practitioners so naturally. Based on the exploration of similarities between these two professional worldviews, the anthropological model for child and youth care worker education and practice has been formulated.

The special relationship described above should be analyzed against the backdrop of negative or even hostile attitudes toward researchers that prevailed in the setting. These are widely shared by members of the child and youth care work community (see Beker & Baizerman 1982; Garduque & Peters, 1982; VanderVen, 1993). I learned about these residual feelings only inadvertently, from informal conversations with workers. Later I found out that some of these attitudes were transmitted from one generation of practitioners to the next as part of the peer-socialization process. The stereotypes persisted in spite of high staff turnover.

Located in the vicinity of several university and college campuses in a large metropolitan area, the setting served as a popular practicum placement for students in the human service professions. Its staff had ongoing involvement with various representatives of academia and tended to view research activities as investigator-oriented: "Those academics use the institution to satisfy their curiosity." Their endeavors were regarded as exploitative and were often referred to as "hit-and-run" activities. "They come, or just send their assistants, have their questionnaires filled out, and vanish."

One frequent complaint concerned the applicability of findings: "They don't care about our problems. Do they have to stay here and struggle with the everyday reality of working with kids?" Another pertained to the process of researchers feeding back their findings to the organization: "That is, when they bother to let us know about them [the findings] at all. Mostly they end up sending a brief report or a copy of some journal article, months or even years later. That, too, is kept up in the office. Never mind the time *we* wasted on the stupid project."

Encounters with representatives of the evaluation research world seldom constituted positive experiences for these workers, either. Although topics may have been more relevant, these researchers' presence usually connoted change and control. They tended to be called in by the administrative echelons "when things were not going all that well." Cooperation with outside evaluators entailed answering probing questions, often without satisfactory assurances for safeguarding anonymity. Furthermore, workers were aware that the "implementation of findings," whatever those might be, meant departure from their accustomed ways of doing things, which was inherently threatening.

Practitioners spend long hours with the residents and come to see the world from their perspective. This is an asset in that it enables them to form trusting and lasting relationships with their charges. At the same time it evokes in them antagonism toward a generalized, blanket category of "outsiders" that, in addition to researchers, includes representatives of various social welfare and counseling service organizations. What all these outsiders are considered to have in common is membership in groups invested with decision-making power over the future of young people whom only they, the direct care workers, claim to truly know (Durkin, 1990).

ANTHROPOLOGISTS AND CHILD AND YOUTH CARE WORKERS

A comparison of the anthropologist's working style and way of reasoning in the traditional context of studying small scale tribal societies with the style and reasoning of child and youth care workers follows.

Anthropological Thinking in Cross-Paradigm Perspective

Anthropologists have traditionally done fieldwork in "exotic" societies about which little, if any, systematic knowledge was available. In order to come to understand their culture, the anthropologist had to piece together a mosaic of their life ways through a meticulous process of information gathering. This genre of research favors the mapping of an entire cultural unit–or, in anthropological terms, adopts a holistic approach to topics studied–before proceeding to the in-depth study of distinctive domains (Dobbert, 1982; Wolcott, 1990). This is quite different from the more common route taken by social scientists working within the neopositivist paradigm (Kerlinger, 1989; Newman, 1994) who study various aspects of their own society. Based on a working knowledge of the culture, they can use standardized instruments or methods and are able to formulate or test hypotheses concerning focused research interests.

Neopositivist social researchers and anthropologists also use different criteria for evaluating the nature of scientific truth. While the former look for an absolute and objective TRUTH, verifiable and replicable given the use of the "proper" scientific methods, the latter's interest lies in uncovering the multiplicity of their informants' subjective "truths," which are believed to be rooted in these individuals' personal and cultural histories.

Different value orientations toward the populations studied guide investigators within these two research paradigms. Those following the neopositivist tradition maintain a stance of affective neutrality and view themselves as outsiders to their research ventures. Anthropologists, on the other hand, consider themselves immersed in their studies and recognize their influence on and commitment to its results. All documented positions expressed by informants are accepted as "legitimate"; the ethnographer's role is to record them and attempt to understand or interpret them within their own cultural context.

The experience acquired through working with foreign cultures makes anthropologists respectful of diversity. Cross-cultural wisdom has taught them that there are different ways to achieve similar or equivalent goals, none more valid than the other by absolute or universal standards. These are regarded as adaptive strategies devised by people to suit their needs. In other words, ethnographic fieldworkers embrace a stance of cultural relativism.

The fieldwork experience. The ability to ask pertinent questions is believed to develop in the course of long term, intimate association with the members of a culture, through learning the local language, basic life routines, the group's social structure, and the meanings attributed to cultural events. This intimate involvement is expected to socialize the fieldworker to do and see things the local way. In other words, how an anthropologist thinks and the questions he or she asks are, to a great extent, determined by the historical circumstances under which the "pioneers" of the profession carried out their fieldwork. The attitudes formed in that process left their imprint on the philosophy of the discipline and the professional ethics of its practitioners.

The ethnographer assumes the stance of the culture learner guided by the "natives" throughout the exploration. Knowledge is acquired through the eclectic use of a number of research tools, such as participant observation, in-depth interviewing, and the collection of life histories. To obtain a variety of insiders' viewpoints on a cultural phenomenon and also as a validity check on the fieldworker's own insights, a large number of informants representing different social positions are contacted. These interviews yield a multi-layered cultural narrative.

Life in the field also teaches ethnographers to diagnose their personal biases, record their own feelings and distinguish between the descriptive, analytic, and interpretive layers of their inquiry (Wolcott, 1994). By so doing, they become sensitive, self-aware human research instruments.

Culture: Ecological and cognitive definitions. Culture, anthropology's seminal concept, has been given numerous definitions.[1] I bring here two definitions that are instrumental for developing an anthropological approach to child and youth care work. From an ecological standpoint, culture is an adaptive mechanism

1. See Kroeber and Kluckhohn, 1952, and Kaplan and Manners, 1972, for classical discussions of the culture concept, and Spindler and Spindler, 1990, for a more recent one.

that a population develops over time to adjust to its physical–or material–and social environment. From a cognitive stance, a group's culture can be envisioned as a set of rules, norms, and values, or a mental road map to follow (Spradley, 1972).

While the ecological definition links the notion of culture to a territory, the cognitive one places it in people's heads. Knowledge becomes the stuff of culture, and a group of people with such shared knowledge–a culture. This distinction helps clarify why any human collective's way of life becomes accessible to people who were not born into it only as a system of ideas they can learn.

Cognitive cultures and their members. The emphasis on knowledge makes it possible to conceive of professional groups, such as physicians, teachers, and child care workers, and of organizations and their subsystems, like hospitals and wards, schools and classrooms, day and residential treatment centers and cottages within them, and even of families as cultural units. They each have exclusive knowledge, overt and covert symbols, a unique structure, and rules for new members to join. A cultural approach to small groups justifies the use of anthropological theory and methods for their analysis.

Membership in such cognitive cultures entails the assumption of several identities simultaneously. For example, adults may have a professional, a political, and a family identity, to name only a few. Youngsters may have one identity in the classroom, a second in their peer-group culture, and a third in their family context. Youth in residential care are likely to have even more cultural affiliations. The ability to manage these memberships becomes a measure of one's adaptation in complex, modern societies. In certain cases there is a consonance in norms and values between these reference groups. For instance, a young married male physician counts on his family to accept his long absences and to support the intensive time investment in his career during his residency years, in the hope of trade-offs from his professional success in the future.

However, people are often expected to function in contexts with discrepant demands. Young people in residential care are likely to belong to the latter category, with potential tension among program, peer group, and family expectations. This is equally true of child and youth care workers, who are also torn between the dictates of clashing identities that demand full availability for emotionally charged work with clients (Maier, 1990) and long shifts that keep them away from their families yet leave them with the frustration and financial burden of an insufficiently remunerated job (Ferguson, 1993). The situation is often further complicated by workers' attempts to pursue academic studies in child and youth care concomitantly with their work (Ferguson, 1990).

The culture of child and youth care organizations. The residential treatment center as well as other child and youth care settings can be considered as cultures from both an ecological and cognitive standpoint. Territorially bounded, their mandate is derived from needs created by the larger cultural system of which they are a part. Their social mission is accomplished, at least in part, through the purposive design of their environment.

At the same time such organizations constitute cognitive cultural units with norms, values, social structures, symbol systems, and languages of their own. They can be subdivided into smaller entities based on members' organizational or professional reference groups. According to the anthropological paradigm, all members of this culture–clients, child care workers, clinical staff, consultative and administrative staff, maintenance workers–are treated as informants without whom the study would not have been possible, rather than as "subjects." Only through their willing cooperation can the investigator gain access to the kind of in-depth information that he or she seeks.

Transactions of meanings are at the core of all social interaction. This underscores the importance of uncovering the meaning-attribution processes operant in child and youth care settings, which are dynamic, negotiated systems based on the various inputs of their participants. Keeping this multiplicity distinctly in mind at all times is a formidable task.

Nevertheless, much like other small-scale cultures, these organizations tend to be intolerant of deviance because it threatens the integrity of their social fabric. They commonly uphold a normative ethos. Bringing about change in clients in clearly defined, often behaviorally specified ways is considered the *raison d'être* of many of these organizations. In the light of this and given the reality of multicultural client populations, highlighting the importance of cultural diversity in such environments cannot be overemphasized.

The degree of inclusiveness or exclusiveness of any definition of culture is established as a matter of convention among members of the community who share the definition. In other words, a child and youth care setting, residential or non-residential, can be treated as a cultural unit in and of itself when interest lies in analyzing its internal dynamics, interactive patterns, or climate. However, a more comprehensive definition will include the whole of the child and youth care service delivery field: policy makers, funding sources, socializing agents and institutions, and professional groups and their ideologies.

CULTURAL LEARNING THEORY

Cognitive and Interpersonal Approaches

Most studies of cultural learning draw an analytic distinction between people and their culture. Enculturation theory underlying these studies posits that learners absorb knowledge passively. Based on the analysis of ethnographic literature, Spindler (1975) offers a descriptive model of the mechanisms of culture transmission operant in the societies he has sampled. In this early but influential formulation (see Spindler, 1987, for a later position on this matter) he portrays the induction of neophytes into their culture as an interpersonal process.

According to this conceptualization, mechanisms of cultural "compression" and "decompression" are alternated in the process of socializing new members. Compression is expressed through the imposition of strict limitations on the initiate's socially approved behavioral options, until he or she can exhibit mastery of the rules of proper conduct. This is followed by a period of decompression, or a broadening of the acceptable behavioral repertoire, along with the allocation of social rights and responsibilities. This dialectic model envisions individuals' progress from one of these role-learning contexts to the other as a compressive-decompressive cycle.

Gearing (1974) perceives cultural transmission/acquisition as a dynamic process of information flow that takes place in dyadic face-to-face interactions in the course of which "equivalences of meaning" are transacted between learners and socializing agents. Learning on both sides occurs as a result of post-encounter assessments of the parties' expectations or "agendas." While allotting an active part to learners, this model focuses on the social aspects of the process and disregards the environment as a source of learning. For this reason, these cognitive approaches cannot be considered holistic theories.

A Holistic Dynamic Approach

Over the last two decades a cross-cultural research team of educational anthropologists, of which I was a member, formulated and tested a theory of cultural learning (Dobbert, 1975; Dobbert & Eisikovits, 1984; Pitman, Eisikovits & Dobbert, 1989) based on a broad and dynamic definition of culture. This conceptualization includes both cognitive and ecological-materialist dimensions. It allows for continuous assessment of the correspondence between a group's life way and its environment.

Members of all human collectives, regardless of their age and social status, learn continuously, both consciously and unconsciously: (a) appropriate styles of participation in ever-changing interactions; (b) how to perform new tasks; and (c) how to fulfill new roles. People generalize from their experience and by so doing shape their future acts and encounters. Through their interpretation of existing codes and performance based on these interpretations, members preserve some cultural features while changing others.

Significant learning takes place due to learners' exposure to their environment, such as the manipulation of objects and participation in the operation of various social institutions, e.g., learning appropriate behavioral patterns through going to church, buying in a supermarket, using an instant cash machine or a soft drink vendor. The dual emphasis on the culture acquisition potential inherent in interaction with human agents as well as material structures and objects illustrates the holistic and dynamic nature of this theory.

Separation between people and cultural patterns is viewed as arbitrary. Instead, learners are treated as integral to the socio-cultural patterns they attempt to acquire–that is, as active agents who select options while they learn from a variety of social and physical sources through different sensory channels. This non-linear modality of culture acquisition is due to the polyphasic nature of human learning (Henry, 1960), which means that at any given moment a number of inputs are processed simultaneously.

The ability to influence this natural process via deliberate intervention is limited. Social agents–such as parents, teachers, and child and youth care workers–and institutions–like families, schools, and child and youth care agencies–do a significant amount of directing and teaching of the young in the course of their transformation into "desirable" adults. According to this broad conceptualization, however, all participants are at the same time learners and designers of their culture, which is perennially modified by members' acts and interactions.

Having established that child and youth care organizations are cultures in both the ecological and cognitive sense of the term makes them amenable to ethnographic study and cultural analysis. The following section illustrates possibilities for applying this model to better understand life in such settings.

CULTURAL LEARNING IN CHILD AND YOUTH CARE CONTEXTS

Child and youth care settings provide conditions that foster active learning and emphasize the receiving rather than the transmitting end of the continuum (Hansen, 1982; Pitman, Eisikovits, & Dobbert, 1989; Wolcott, 1982). Practitioners are facilitators of this cultural learning process. "Culture acquisition" or "cultural learning" is the umbrella concept. It includes both "schooling" as the narrowest and most formal type of training and "education" as a larger modality of deliberate instruction that may occur in a variety of contexts. Child and youth care agencies, particularly residential ones, are designed to provide conditions more reminiscent of naturally occurring learning than other educational environments.

Thus, workers are seen as co-creators of the culture of the organization. The implications of such an active perception of their role have to be considered. By highlighting their system-modifying capacity, this model alerts child and youth care work educators in general, and organizers of institution-based training programs in particular, to the limited impact of formal training (Beker & Barnes, 1990). As polyphasic learners (Henry, 1960) these workers are open to many other formative influences. Through informal contacts with peers, interaction with clients, and growing familiarity with the milieu as a whole, they form their own picture of the covert as well as overt dimensions of the system and their own role in it (Grupper & Eisikovits, 1993).

The overall culture of such a setting is also shaped by the dynamic input of clients. Assuming that it is possible to educate through programs, rules, and regulations, as the cognitive theories of cultural learning tend to suggest, is unrealistic. There is ample research evidence to substantiate the incongruence between deliberately transmitted information and knowledge actually internalized in structured classroom situations (Aronowitz & Giroux, 1993; Ogbu, 1987; Vogt, Jordan, & Tharp, 1987; Wilcox, 1982). This is all the more true in holistic child and youth care environments where learners are exposed to a wide range of culture transmitting sources–human and material, structural and processual (Pitman, Eisikovits, & Dobbert, 1989).

In residential contexts, youngsters learn in the kitchen from helping the cook, and they learn from talking to the handyman. They discover discrepancies between stated norms and actual practices and find ways to manipulate the system. To counteract this, it is best to involve them in formulating the rules (Maluccio, 1991).

Adoption of the anthropological model of child and youth care work will help practitioners become change-sensitive, process-oriented observers and analysts and conscious co-designers of the systems within which they function and those with which they interact, such as families, communities, and referral agencies.

THE ANTHROPOLOGICAL MODEL IN ACTION

Jones (1985) argues that residential child care is the seminal form of child and youth care work, indeed the context that shaped its basic tenets. Savicki (1993) calls for the diffusion of these principles to other areas of practice. Because of my own familiarity with the residential care field, I use it for purposes of illustration, but the model is applicable to the rhythm and reality of other services as well.

How does this model contribute to the professional functioning of child and youth care workers? What opportunities do they have to perform ethnographic tasks on the job? Examples follow on three levels: the cottage or unit, the organization, and in inter-organizational levels.

Ethnographic Fieldwork in the Cottage

To attend to the different nuances of meaning underlying interaction in the cottage, practitioners must learn to identify and map the various meaning-sharing groups, their distinctive features, and their modes of interrelating. Therefore, it is suggested that new workers start out as nonparticipant observers until they gain sufficient cultural knowledge to successfully engage in active participation, or spend this time alternating between worker and observer roles. The assistance of more experienced colleagues, with whom beginners are usually teamed up, can be instrumental. Comparing perspectives will prove mutually enriching. Questions and observations from the neophytes as "outsiders" provide fresh insights to the veteran members of the team.

The log, which serves as a written medium of communication among direct care workers in the cottage, can be turned into a reliable data base. Various techniques can be developed as a team effort to assure inter-subjective note-taking. For example, ethnographers often employ field guides and standardized observation sheets to maximize the accuracy of recording. Such guides serve as reminders of the behavioral areas to be covered and the degree of detailed background information and verbatim reproduction of speech patterns desired, particularly in collaborative research projects (Whiting, 1968; Dobbert & Eisikovits, 1984).

In spite of hectic schedules, the cottage routine has built-in time slots for accomplishing such ethnographic tasks. "Quiet time" and night shifts allow for the worker's own note-taking and analysis, for "catching up on cottage news," and for comparing interpretations of residents' behavioral patterns through the log. Team meetings also serve as occasions for oral transactions illuminating meanings and collaborative planning.

Guttmann (1991) suggests that much of what child and youth care workers are called upon to do involves on-the-spot reaction to crisis situations–immediacies–that do not allow time for pre-intervention strategizing. Nevertheless, since practitioners may not have been present at the scene of events when such crises occurred (one would assume that their presence would forestall many such crises), it usually is quite feasible for them to attempt to clarify the occurrence and its antecedents before taking further action, unless they are facing an emergency.

This task is accomplished by soliciting accounts of the events from a large number of participants in order to gain a rounded picture. Even if workers' reactions are later "judged" inappropriate by self, team, or supervisors, they can be corrected in the light of information subsequently gathered. This strategy has the added advantage of providing youths in residential care with a self-reflective model of adult decision making.

Organizational and Inter-Organizational Level Applications

Due to the amount of time devoted to work with clients, a strong cottage identity becomes pervasive among workers. It often outweighs the sense of identification with the institution at large. The cottage and its team become a universe unto themselves. Such a tendency toward closure is exhibited by many human services through the reduction of information exchange with other systems, and it is often expressed in routinization. The holistic view inherent in the anthropological approach helps to counterbalance this. Its application re-establishes the relevance of the institution at large, with its combined educational and treatment philosophy, as the proper frame of reference for effective practice.

A holistic vision is further reinforced by the organizational functions workers fulfill outside the cottage, coordinating between the residents and the various institutional subsystems–such as the school, the recreation department, health care personnel, and the administration–as well as in working with outside agencies. In all these contacts they serve as cultural translators, providing representatives of less directly involved audiences with relevant information about their clients to facilitate communication and intervention.

Anthropology's comparative perspective can also be harnessed to help maintain a broad-angle view. This can be achieved by working out inter-cottage exchange programs for practitioners. Such arrangements carry further organizational advantages. They create an atmosphere of openness and sharing that encourages treating one's experiences as resources from which co-workers can also benefit, particularly when these are documented and systematically recorded. This eases direct care workers' sense of isolation, thereby potentially reducing burnout rates.

The comparative perspective offers a frame of reference for conceptualizing one's everyday experiences in more universalistic categories (Beker, 1989) which, in turn, produces more reflective and innovative workers. This is one possible avenue toward unlocking the "tacit knowledge" of practitioners (Argyris, Putnam, & Smith, 1985; Schon, 1987, 1991).

In sum, the model of child and youth care work presented here presupposes a flexible and self-confident management style that encourages workers to initiate grass-roots change, fosters ongoing assessment of needs, and results in service improvement. To maintain staff motivation, however, administrators have to provide career advancement opportunities and proper remuneration for worker efforts. According to Durkin (1990), investment in upgrading the professional quality of child and youth care workers would prove to be both more cost effective and inherently more advantageous to the field than leaving leadership roles in the hands of other human service professionals.

The anthropological approach can be applied on various organizational levels, as illustrated, or can be focused on individuals or groups of participants, typical interactions, or recurring events. For example, a staff member can follow a client's behavioral patterns in various contexts as a basis for preparing a well-researched evaluation report. A supervisor can observe and analyze workers' performance for educational purposes and feed the findings back to them (Phelan, 1990). The comparative study of professional encounters within different units, such as team meetings or weekly group meetings, helps to establish systematic data bases for use in various evaluation contexts.

ACQUIRING THE MODEL

This model provides practitioners with a particular world-view. Educators in the field may be the first to fully understand the implications of cultural learning theory for the child and youth care system as a whole and for the place of educational and training institutions within it (VanderVen, 1993). Since learning is ongoing, it cannot be neatly sequentionalized into chronologically ordered categories such as "pre-service," "in-service," or "on-the-job" training. It is an integral part of the culture, and formal educational institutions can take responsibility for transmitting only certain aspects of its holistic knowledge base.

However, these educators are the best equipped to sensitize the field to the potential inherent in this approach. Training child and youth care workers to apply the model with simultaneous exposure to theory in cultural and educational anthropology will optimally occur as systematic learning experiences within degree programs. A supervised ethnographic fieldwork experience can serve as the bridge between the formal education (including practicum) and the practice stage of a career in child and youth care work (Pence, 1990). Intensive workshops combined with fieldwork experiences (VanderVen, 1993) can also be effective in achieving some of these objectives.

The application of the theoretical concepts as well as the field methods lend themselves to experiential transmission and acquisition. As illustrated here, child and youth care agencies provide ample opportunities for such experimentation. To achieve the distance necessary for developing the ethnographic stance, however, it is advisable to conduct fieldwork exercises in other settings as well. Thus, performing cultural mappings of a variety of social institutions such as schools, hospitals, churches, prisons, banks, factories, or retail businesses can be beneficial. The comparative study of their languages, symbolic structures, value systems, and social organization illustrates the notion of culturally patterned behavior.

Simultaneous introduction to classical anthropological studies of territorially bounded groups such as tribal societies, religious communities, ethnic enclaves, and street corner gangs promotes a broader understanding of culture theory. Ethnographic films are also potent didactic tools. Discussing these films provides a good context for elucidating ethical dilemmas arising in the field, as well as for studying fieldwork styles and methods.

The model can be adapted to suit the needs of workers with

different educational backgrounds and organizational roles. The ability to use it actively, as opposed to merely "understanding the language," will vary according to one's level of familiarity with its various aspects.

Dissemination should be aimed as widely as possible. Those with active research skills can assume responsibility for such complex activities as planning self-evaluation projects, designing systemic changes, or performing pattern-level data analysis (see Gauthier, 1990). But even passive command of the anthropological language has heuristic value.

Practitioners in this field operate in high intensity environments whose dynamic character often renders planned pre-intervention decision making difficult. The following chapters suggest various ways to overcome this problem and demonstrate the empowering effect of applying this approach in child and youth care work contexts.

Chapter 2

Ethnographic Description as a Vehicle for Child and Youth Care Worker Education

How can descriptive ethnography help child and youth care workers apply this model, thereby enhancing the quality of their work with clients? The following ethnographic account is jargon-free, which makes it accessible. The material is presented from the perspective of a *new girl*[1] and a new *youth counselor*, both of whom are newcomers and have to "learn the ropes." This ethnography concentrates on the overt socialization practices these two categories of neophytes undergo. It does not cover the intricate, day by day polyphasic cultural learning that takes place in the setting among all members, old and new.

The selection presents and compares two parallel processes of formal induction into the culture of the institution. In addition to providing a balanced picture, emphasizing commonalities between clients and workers in this regard highlights the pervasiveness of the phenomenon of staff turnover, which is almost as fast as client turnover. Its effects on the organization also become apparent. Under these circumstances it is hard to envision child and youth care

---

1. Italics are used to highlight local or setting-specific use of language in the particular residential center being described.

[Haworth co-indexing entry note]: "Ethnographic Description as a Vehicle for Child and Youth Care Worker Education." Eisikovits, Rivka A. Co-published simultaneously in *Child & Youth Services* (The Haworth Press, Inc.) Vol. 18, No. 1, 1997, pp. 21-42; and: *The Anthropology of Child and Youth Care Work* (Rivka A. Eisikovits) The Haworth Press, Inc., 1997, pp. 21-42. Single or multiple copies of this article are available from The Haworth Document Delivery Service [1-800-342-9678, 9:00 a.m. - 5:00 p.m. (EST). E-mail address: getinfo@haworth.com].

workers as representatives of the "system." In fact, as a researcher, I found that residents were often more knowledgeable than the direct care workers about life in the center.

Since communication is so important, learning the local language is crucial. That is why I preferred the peer socialization model to present the material. Rather than following the handbook of regulations, which was one of the options, I chose the *big sister* approach (see page 26) to bring out perspectives on cottage life. Both socialization approaches emphasize the centrality of basic routines and the formation of habits of consistent behavior, such as family living skills. Clients' behavioral problems are largely attributed to lack of structure in their home environment.

Values can be voiced, they can appear in written statements, or they can be more subtly built into the program. In this chapter, value consonance among socializing agents and organizational structures is stressed. In Chapter 3, discrepancies between overt values and actual practices become the focus of our attention.

In this selection the normative course of events is laid out. Non-normative, or less preferred options, such as leaving through the "back door" or the "side door" (see pages 33-34) are only briefly mentioned. Also the *youth counselor*'s initial socialization to the culture of the institution is described more briefly than that of the *new girl*, based on the assumption that the former is more familiar to workers. This is not a valid assumption when ethnographic material is meant to serve as a "model" rather than as a "mirror." A more detailed, non-selective style of presentation would have been better suited to the former purpose.

In such a dynamic culture with so many categories of participants whose actions are based on different agendas, it is crucial to apply anthropology's multi-instrument approach (combining participant observation with interviewing and other research methods, including analyzing written documents when they are available) to look at behavior in different contexts longitudinally, so as to compare what participants do with what they say (Spradley, 1980). This will also improve interaction with clients and cooperation within the staff system (Wozner, 1991).

The Cultural Scene of a Juvenile Treatment Center for Girls: Another Look[1]

Alvin Gouldner (1975) distinguishes between the commonly perceived role of sociology to "discover" reality and its other, no less central function, to "display the already known." The potentially dissenting reader will raise two questions concerning the above title:

1. Why bother to take "another look" at a juvenile treatment center for girls and describe an already known entity?
2. What do I mean by "the cultural scene" of a treatment center?

The need for repeated and constant reexamination of treatment centers is dictated by what I consider to be the very essence of such programs: communication. Effective communication, or "meaningful interaction," as it is frequently referred to, can take place only if all the actors involved in a situation are aware of everybody else's perceptions, interpretations, and use of language in that particular situation. In other words, accurate communication is contingent upon shared meaning. But is it fair to assume that meanings, once captured, can be safely considered to be "already known?" Do meanings not change? They most certainly do. In any given setting, the redefinition of meanings is an ongoing process that occurs weekly, daily, even hourly, and it is further enhanced by the frequent changes of actors. Therefore, in order to maintain good commication in treatment centers, a prerequisite for good treatment, child care workers must relentlessly keep up with these changes of meanings by continuing to reexamine and recheck the "already known."

There is yet another reason why I consider it beneficial for the child and youth care worker to read about other treatment centers. I think that a short episode will help to clarify my point. While I was doing fieldwork in the treatment center I am about to describe, I was working in the setting as a part-time youth counselor and

---

1. This selection is adapted from R. A. Eisikovits, "The Cultural Scene of a Juvenile Treatment Center for Girls: Another Look," *Child Care Quarterly, 9*(3), 1980, with the permission of the editor and Human Sciences Press.

communication consultant. During our weekly team meetings I would take a few minutes to read some of my notes to the team members for corrections and feedback. Here are some of the typical reactions:

- Is this really what we sound like?
- Could all this make sense to an outsider?
- Isn't that ridiculous, how much time we spent on her?
- He was speaking all the time, making all the decisions.

Gradually, they started using my field notes to evaluate their group process. These both stimulated them and provided that minimal distance necessary to contemplate their own actions. I hope that child care workers can achieve a similar distancing by reading a description of another treatment center, possibly very much like their own, possibly not, and that the following account will enable them to take that relaxed, reflective, dispassionate look of the outsider at some of the same problems they may be facing in their own settings.

I now borrow the anthropologist's perspective to explain the concept of the "cultural scene of a treatment center." I shall pretend to set out on an expedition to study and report on a foreign culture I know nothing about, and I realize that in order to get a complete and accurate picture of that culture I need to check and recheck every detail with appropriate informants. If my expedition is successful, I expect to return from this imaginary journey with a new metaphor: The treatment center as a culture with a language, norms, values, and a social and political structure of its own.

THE PHYSICAL SETTING

Springdale[2] is located in a suburban residential area, surrounded by a large, green, open space and lined by a long wooded stretch on the west and a private lake on the north. The complex is divided into three main parts connected by tunnels for easy winter accessibility. In the south wing of the main building are the administration, social

2. All names of settings and of people appearing in this volume are fictitious.

services, and conference rooms. The same wing houses a public school that offers a special education program for the junior and senior high school age residents as well as for day students with learning disabilities from the surrounding community. The food service, cafeteria, laundry, and maintenance departments are in the basement of the south wing. A day care program serving some 30 neighborhood preschoolers is also located on the lower level of this building. It offers part-time jobs for residents interested in learning more about child care.

Five small buildings called *cottages*, housing 12 residents each, are located to the east of the main building. The girls have separate rooms. The cottages are decorated in warm, lively colors with comfortable furniture, a fireplace, lounge areas, color TV, stereo systems, and so on, which create a home-like atmosphere.

The following account describes a *new girl*'s experience of becoming a resident. The participants are introduced here in the actual order in which she meets and begins to interact with them. Subsequently, a new treatment staff member, called a *youth counselor* is described on his way into the system. The description portrays the widening scope of the *new girl*'s and the new *youth counselor*'s cultural knowledge of the *Center*. In the process a complete picture of the setting as a cultural entity unfolds.

BECOMING A RESIDENT

The *new girl* becomes acquainted with the setting during an initial interview called *intake*. The residential treatment center serves adolescent girls between the ages of 12-18–some committed by the court, some referred by other social service agencies, with a range of behavioral and emotional problems. The participants in this encounter, in addition to the girl herself, are representatives of the referring agency (juvenile court, probation officer, county welfare, etc.) and sometimes a family member. The center is represented by the intake worker and the *cottage* social worker whose role becomes gradually clearer to the *new girl*, from here on called Joan.

The *intake worker* starts out by describing the program. She explains the basis of *cottage* living, emphasizes that all *girls* have to consent to their placement, which means that they agree to cooperate with the treatment staff in working on their problems. Then all participants proceed to map out the major areas Joan will work on at Springdale. Either before or after *intake*, the social worker gives Joan a tour of the school and the *cottage*. She learns that the average length of stay is nine months and also that it is up to her to complete the program sooner if she can. After intake, Joan is to stay for a one-week trial period in one of the *cottages*. "At that point (when the trial week is over), we'll have a meeting with you and the *cottage team* to see how things are working out and to decide if this is the right place for you," says the *intake worker,* concluding the first encounter.

In the *cottage* Joan is greeted by the same social worker, a *youth counselor* and the *girls*. Sally, one of the *old girls,* is assigned to be her *big sister*. She shows Joan around and tries to maker her feel at home. The *big sister* volunteers to spend more time with the *new girl* during the first few weeks until she makes friends with others in the group.

Two of the *cottages* use short handbooks instead of *big sisters* to lay out the daily routine and basic expectations. In these *cottages,* every *new girl* gets a copy, and a *youth counselor* goes over it with her. I chose to follow the *big sister* model for several reasons. First, it is the one used in the *cottage* where I did most of my observation. Second, it gives an idea of how the peer group is used as an integral part of the program. The program emphasizes verbal interaction; the improvement of communication skills, to facilitate this interaction, is a high priority. Thus, Sally's command of language as an *old girl*, when compared to that of a *new girl*'s is striking.

The following dialogue calls the reader's attention to the large amount of new vocabulary and concepts a *new girl* needs to learn in the process of becoming a resident. The exact meaning of italicized words is different in the setting from their use outside and, as such, is new for Joan. Sally shows Joan her room. On the stairs she tells her: "We are not supposed to smoke or eat upstairs. These are the two big *No's* upstairs." On the door of Joan's room they spot a colorful sign with the inscription, "WELCOME JOAN." Sally stays with Joan while she unpacks and the two start talking:

S: Where do I start?

J: I don't know . . . Tell me what it's like.

S: Relax, it's not a bad place. Anyway, let me tell you how things work around here. On school days you get up at 7:00 o'clock. *Night staff* wakes you up. At 7:30 we have breakfast. Everybody is supposed to be at breakfast dressed.

J: Who cooks breakfast?

S: We take turns. It's one of the *charges*.

J: One of the what?

S: *Charges*. We all have *charges* around here, you know, to keep the place in shape. If you have *breakfast charge,* you also set the table.

J: Then what?

S: Then we leave for school. First we pick up our rooms a little so it won't be a mess when we get back. School starts at 8:30.

J: What's it like?

S: OK, I guess. Looks like the teachers kind of care about how you're doing. There is about seven or eight kids in each class and we get to choose our topics. Work on them as long as we want. If you're behind on credits, its real easy to make them up here. I never thought I'd catch up in my old school, you know.

J: No Shit!

S: They also give you jobs, you know, after you've been here for a while. You can get out for a few hours everyday and be like a teacher's aide or something. Work with little kids, all sorts of things. You get credit for it, and it's good money, too.

J: No shit!

S: You have to prove yourself first, though. And if you run you lose your job.

J: No shit!

S: You can't smoke either, only at lunch time in the cafeteria. During breaks. Some kids smoke in the bathroom, though. But they get caught a lot. I'm kind of getting used to it now, but it was hard at first.

J: Shit!

S: Anyway . . . we get back from school at 2:00 in the afternoon. Sit around and chat for a while, then we have *school group* around 2:30.

J: What's *school group?*

S: Just sitting at the table with a *staff.* Talking about how the day went in school and all that. *Staff* goes over the memos. If you have a bad *memo* . . .

J: A *memo?*

S: Took me a while, too, until I had it figured out. Anyway, *memos,* let's say you did something wrong during Math, so the teacher writes a bad *memo* to the *cottage staff* to tell them about it. But you can get good *memos,* too, if you're doing good in class. Sometime you need to bug them a little about the good *memos*. They never forget to write the bad ones.

J: I bet they don't.

S: One of the teachers is in charge of the *girls* in our *cottage* when they're in school. She brings over the *memos* after school to our *staff.* We get to keep a copy for our *personal log*.

J: How's that?

S: Each *girl* has a notebook with her name on it. Every night the *staff* write in it how you're doing, what you need to work on, stuff like that. The *logs* are in the office but you can read them if you want to.

J: You do, eh?

S: *School group* only takes like 30 minutes or something. You can snack or smoke if you want to. Then we get some time to go for a walk down to the lake or ride the horses or play tennis. You can also play ping-pong or pool in the basement if you want to.

J: What horses?

S: Haven't seen them? There are four horses here and each *cottage* has a riding day. You can ride around the trails.

J: When can I do that?

S: First you have to have Sue, the recreation director, ride with you. Tomorrow is our day so I'll take you. After a couple of lessons you get your privileges and can ride by yourself.

J: Wow!

S: At 4:00 we have our *regular group*.

J: *Regular group?*

S: You know, the kind where we sit in a circle, and talk about everybody's problems and how you deal with them. Try to give people feedback. Or if there's any hassle with someone in the *cottage* we try to work it out in *group*. In our *cottage* we can sit on the carpet during *group* and smoke. See you're not supposed to smoke on the good furniture, like the sofa and the armchairs. But in some of the *cottages* they sit on chairs and can't smoke during *group* at all.

J: Shit.

S: We're kind of lucky. Anyway, *group* takes about an hour. Then it's dinnertime. We eat at 5:30. If you have *dining room charge* you set the table and pick up the trays from the kitchen. You have to have a *staff* with you.

J: Why?

S: Pretty dumb. So you don't drop dinner, I guess. We say Grace and all and if you want to pray for somebody special that day, you can mention it, too. After dinner we rinse our plates and if you have *kitchen charge,* you put everything away and load the dishwasher. Kitchen is a lousy *charge,* but you only have it like every six weeks.

J: That's plenty.

S: After dinner you can smoke a cigarette and then we all go up to our rooms for *quiet hour.*

J: Can't speak for a whole hour?!

S: What it means is that you kind of relax, or read a book, or write letters, or do some schoolwork, things like that.

J: What d'you do after that?

S: We come down and there's always something going on. One evening we go swimming or we go bowling. Most of the time we have some activity out here. If there's a good show, you can watch it. We get to plan out the activities for the month with the *staff.* See there on the wall? That's our calendar of events.

J: Tell me something else. That *girl,* I don't know her name, she's talking on the phone. Can you call from here?

S: I am sure the *staff* will explain that one, but anyway, we have phone rules. *New girls* can only call their family. Later on you can call some of your friends if you want to, but you have to *request* it in *team* to put them on the *phone list* so they can be okayed by your family and the *staff* first. You know, to make sure you don't talk to people who have bad influence on you.

J: Never heard about *team requests*.

S: Quite an event around here. It's on Wednesdays and all the *staff* are here for it and all. First they have a meeting to talk about us and how we were doing that week. Then we have a big *group* with all the *girls* and all the team. Team means when all the *staff* are here together.

J: You call them *youth counselors,* no? What are they like?

S: They're OK, I guess. You kind of get to like them. We call everybody *staff,* but they call themselves *youth counselors*. They help you work out problems with your family. We go for walks or canoeing on the lake for *one-to-ones*. I get along pretty good with most of them. You have a *special staff* who takes you shopping when you need something. Like every two *girls* have the same *shopper.*

J: *One-to-ones?*

S: Oh, it just means when we spend time alone with a *staff,* we get into heavy stuff, like talk about things that are on our *treatment plan,* or you can just have a good time together.

J: I think I have an idea what *treatment plan* is. At intake they sort of told me about that.

S: Don't worry, the *staff* will tell you all about it over and over.

J: Say, do you think I can go home this weekend?

S: Not so fast! You have to be here for two Wednesdays before you can ask for a *team request*.

J: What did you say a *team request* is?

S: In *team request group* the *girls* share how their week went at school, in the *cottage,* how they got along with everybody and usually ask for things like going home to visit for the weekend or to add somebody to their *phone list*.

J: Can you go for the whole weekend?

S: *New girls* go for a few hours. Later you can stay for an *overnight,* then when you've been here for a while and you're doing okay, *working on your goals,* you can stay for the whole weekend.

J: Do you go every week?

S: It depends. Most *girls* only go twice a month. *Older girls* can go three weekends. When you're on *pre-release* you can go every weekend.

J: Is that when you're getting ready to leave?

S: Yeah.

J: What time d'you go to bed?

S: At 11:00. But first you do *charges* at 9:00. See the bulletin board over there? It also explains what exactly you have to do for every *charge.* You do it for a week and then rotate. Once a week you do *super charge* and on Thursdays we have *dorm day,* to clean our rooms, change the towels and sheets and that kind of stuff.

J: You sure do a lot of cleaning around here.

S: It gets pretty messy, you know, and people don't pick up their stuff. So if you don't want to sit in a pit, you need to do something about it. I kind of hate my room when it's a mess.

J: Yeah, me too.

S: After *charges* we go upstairs at 10:00. It takes an hour to get ready for bed. At 11:00 the *night staff* comes up to say goodnight and to turn off the lights.

J: How about the weekends?

S: You can stay up till midnight or you can even watch the late night show, if you want to. Well, I guess I have to get going. I have *dinner charge* this week. Anyway, this kind of wraps it up. Take it easy. I'll be seeing you around.

THE TREATMENT PLAN

During the first week, Joan's cultural circle starts widening. She gets to know all the *girls* in the *cottage* and all the *youth counselors*, the teachers in school, the *girls* from the other *cottages*. If she, or members of her family, have problems with the use of chemicals, she is introduced to the drug counselor. Another colorful figure she meets is the nurse, known to all at Springdale as Ma. Although Ma calls everybody "angel" and listens carefully to "whatever happens to hurt at any particular moment," she "won't be conned easily" or "convert the infirmary into a hiding place from school and other duties."

After two or three weeks of settling in, it is assumed that time is ripe for Joan to start working on her program. The *cottage social worker*, one or two *youth counselors* and Joan herself draw up a tentative *treatment plan*, interpreted as an operational individual growth plan. They list problem areas as are seen by Joan, and formulate them almost entirely in her own words. They set concrete *goals* to eliminate the problems. The staff help her specify the persons who will work with her to achieve each *goal*. This person may be a particular *youth counselor*, the entire *treatment staff* in the *cottage*, a certain friend, but mostly it is Joan herself. A copy of the *treatment plan* is placed in her *personal log*.

This initial *treatment plan* is revised after three months during an encounter known in the setting as *treatment plan review*. When either the *staff* or Joan no longer see certain areas as problematic, they are dropped from the initial plan. New items may occasionally replace them, but this is not interpreted to mean that growth has not occurred. A general rule is that no item is placed on the treatment plan unless Joan herself recognizes it as a problem.

As she progresses through the program from *initial* to *pre-release treatment plan*, Joan enjoys more privileges, such as walking off grounds, usually a job in school, more responsibilities, and also enhanced status in the *cottage*. During the next encounter, the six month review, if she is doing well, her *pre-release treatment plan* is drawn up and gradual reinvolvement in her home community begins. At this stage she usually attends an outside school, participates in its activities, and goes on frequent home visits if her family works closely with the staff of the center.

Family involvement is seen as an essential part of the program. *Cottage* social workers hold bi-weekly individual family sessions in which the *girl* and her family try to "find positive ways of handling conflicts and learn to listen to each other more carefully," in the hope that this will result in overall improved communication. From now on, Joan's widening cultural circle includes the *aftercare worker*, who will be directly involved in her program. Joan will start attending weekly *pre-release groups* with *girls* from all the cottages who are at a similar stage in their program. If the family situation allows it, the *goal* is to prepare her for returning home. If not, the *cottage social worker* and *after-care worker* will help the referring agency find the most suitable alternative for her, such as a group home or a foster home.

When Joan successfully completes her program, the *girls* and *staff* hold a festive graduation ceremony for her, followed by a party in the *cottage* to mark the occasion. Family, friends, *team members,* and other intimates are invited. One of her friends is appointed mistress of ceremonies and is responsible to make sure that everything happens according to plan. This usually includes short speeches by favorite staff members and one or two best friends from the *cottage* about what Joan's presence meant to them and how she helped them *grow.* A few artistic interludes, such as songs or poems are also included.

Says one *cottage social worker*: "Leaving with a party is leaving through the front door." It sometimes happens that *girls* choose to "exit through the back door," that is, to run away. In most cases they are accepted back. This policy is in line with Springdale philosophy that considers patience and perseverance to be synonymous with *caring.* "Leaving through the side door" is yet another alternative, usually resorted to for other than treatment considerations, in such cases as when it is a county's policy to pay for residential treatment up to a maximum length of time irrespective of individual circumstances.

BECOMING A YOUTH COUNSELOR

I shall now describe the socialization process of a *youth counselor* whom I shall call Mike. Like Joan's, his preliminary contact with the

Center is established through an interview. The actors who represent the institution in this encounter are the *administrator,* or at times the entire *administrative team* that includes the *program director,* the *social service supervisor,* and the *youth counselor supervisor.* In the course of this encounter they exchange views on child care philosophy and on the counselor's role in working with children with emotional problems, and they reach agreement in principle that "we are a good place for you and you are a suitable person for us."

Following this, Mike interviews with the *cottage team,* made up of six *youth counselors* and the *cottage social worker.* In this encounter the discussion is on a more concrete level, aimed at checking out personality compatibilities, agreement on ways to make the overall treatment philosophy operative, etc. If the outcome of this interview is also favorable, Mike is hired and his overt socialization begins.

The first two weeks, or *orientation,* constitutes a period of intensive learning and adaptation, during which Mike is supposed to acquire a general familiarity with the setting. Upon completing it, he is expected to be able to act in a culture-appropriate way in most circumstances. During this time he spends the mornings in meetings with heads of various departments, who explain to him how their particular units fit into the overall program and the kinds of responsibilities he will have. He has a long meeting with the *administrator,* who takes the time to explain to him, in a relaxed atmosphere, the essentials of the *treatment philosophy.* Mike spends his afternoons in the *cottage,* observing. Just as Sally, the *big sister,* acquainted Joan with the daily routine of the *cottage,* so does the *cottage supervisor* introduce Mike to his daily work. Mike spends much of his time "getting to know the *girls.*"

During the first few days, Mike is overwhelmed with new information. To help clarify things and serve as an aid to his memory, he receives a file with *orientation* materials. It includes various forms he will have to handle as part of his duties and a "Basic Reading List for Youth Counselors."

During the first six months of his work, Mike participates in a series of on-the-job training sessions conducted by experienced *treatment staff* on topics such as "Being a Team Member," "Treatment Plans and Reviews," "Groups," "Drugs," "Entrance, Release, and Aftercare," "Community Resources," etc. The *youth counselor*'s education continues at a less intensive pace through monthly in-service training sessions devoted to issues of current interest and through outside workshops. The weekly or bi-weekly *supervisory meetings* between the *youth counselor* and the *cottage supervisor* are regarded as a further means of continuing education.

While Joan's acquisition of cultural knowledge takes a centrifugal course, Mike's follows a centripetal one. The *girl* is systematically introduced to *cottage* life and gradually expands her cultural circle to include the rest of the actors in the setting. The *youth counselor* is systematically acquainted with the wider circle first, then anchors his cultural identity in the inner circle of the *cottage* through becoming a *team member.*

THE BELIEF SYSTEM

Now that we have followed two neophytes, a *new girl* and a new *youth counselor,* on their way into the system, let's make sure we understand the major values underlying action in this culture. *Growing* or fostering growth is regarded as a supreme value in the setting. More specifically, the first is what the girls are expected to do and the second is what the environment should do to help them. It is hoped that such growth will occur in the *girl*'s awareness of herself, that is, her ability to identify her own behavioral problems and the reasons underlying them, and consequently, the ways in which she should deal with them in a socially acceptable manner.

Growing as a focal value applies to the treatment staff as well. Manifestations of growth are an enhanced ability to relate to residents and to co-workers, and a general dedication to Springdale and its philosophy.

The *Center* considers it its duty to encourage the professional development of its employees by providing them with various educational opportunities and by using a policy of internal promotion. Metaphorically speaking, one can say that the institution is applying the value of *growing* to its organizational life through diversifying its program and thereby offering a greater variety of services to the community and more opportunities to its staff. An atmosphere of freedom and openness are regarded as necessary means to this desired end. "The *administration,*" says the *program director,* "believes in giving units sufficient freedom to encourage people to try out new things. At the same time, if they have problems that can't be solved within the unit, people should feel both free and open enough to come to the *administration* to discuss them."

Teaching through personal example is another value translated into professional social science terminology as role modeling. The treatment personnel are expected to serve as positive adult role models for the *girls.* Many of the *girls'* problems are believed to stem from a lack of exposure to appropriately functioning adults in their immediate social environment. This explains why the presence of male staff members is considered to be so important.

The belief system emphasizes the importance of building relationships both as a means to the end of *growing* and as an end in itself. Major tools for achieving these *goals* are the encounters where members of the local culture–*girls*, *youth counselors*, *cottage social workers*–exchange and negotiate their perceptions of various situations and interactions. Let's consider some of them.

ENCOUNTERS

Formal Groups

Groups are major tools for social education and individual growth. They provide a reliable support mechanism for resolving conflicts that arise from the group living situation. This is what one of the girls has to say on the subject:

> Sometimes it is boring to sit there for an hour but sometimes you get up feeling easier than when you sat down in the first place. You don't feel like such a creep when you see that other people have the same problems you do. You hear new ideas that worked for other kids.

Some group sessions are devoted to special topics, such as sexuality or drugs, while others are open.

The Team and the Team Meeting

One of the first lessons Mike learns at Springdale concerns his dual role definition as a *youth counselor* and as a *team member.* During the first on-the-job training session devoted to this subject, the *youth counselor supervisor* explains:

> This is a residential treatment center where we need twenty-four hour *staff* coverage seven days a week. To do this each *cottage* has to have six *staff* people. When one *youth counselor* comes on duty, he or she has to know exactly where the other one left off or else we may as well send the kids home, because we clearly can't help them.

The *team* plans the treatment of the *girls.* Its members are accountable to each other for carrying it out accordingly. The *youth counselor supervisor* continues:

> If the *girls* see that you as a *team* are not together, they start manipulating you, trying to play one *counselor* against the other. They'll soon tell you, "But Cathy lets me do it this way, how come you don't?"
>
> The *program director*'s view is, "The *teams* are the most powerful treatment tool we have." This is why they enjoy considerable freedom of action within the framework of the overall philosophy and organizational policies.

Team spirit is believed to depend on efficient communication. Two vehicles designed to assure the proper flow of information among team members are the log, a written medium, and the report, an oral one. Group mood, messages, and major events that occur during the shift are recorded in the general log. Thus, when a counselor comes on duty after an absence of a few days from the setting, he or she should be able to be "filled in" by reading what is recorded in the log for those days. The counselor who goes off duty complements the log by an oral report he or she gives to the colleague who is coming on duty instead.

The *cottage supervisor* believes that "the *girls* do need to see us act as individuals, but they also need to see us operate as a group." The *team's* decision-making processes are seen as models for the *girls'* group interaction. To this end, the *team* often discusses problems related to the *girls* in front of them. *Team members* voice a variety of opinions and give different interpretations of the same behavior. This exposure is considered to be an important educational experience. As one learns from their stories, for many of the *girls,* "This is the first time I see grown-ups who admit they don't always have all the answers." According to one *team member*: "This makes it easier for them to speak up in a *group*. They feel it's okay to be wrong at times and are not afraid to try." The message of modeling their own *group* interaction on the *team meeting* certainly does get across. The *girls* often refer jokingly to the *team meeting* as: "Our *staff* are having *group* now. They have problems to work out, too . . . "

Wednesdays are *team meeting* days. At this time all treatment personnel are present. A considerable part of the agenda is taken up by passing out various information related to personnel policy and other administrative matters, either directly by a representative of the *administration* or indirectly through the *cottage supervisor,* who serves as a liaison between the *administration* and the *teams*. Department heads come into the *team meetings* to explain new procedures related to their units or to ask for their opinions on projected plans. This is an expression of the consensus in the setting that good coordination between *cottage* activities and those of the various departments, such as the recreation department or aftercare, is a major condition for a successful program.

The school liaison is responsible to update the *team* on the *girls'* progress in school during the week. Each *cottage* has a teacher assigned to this task who makes sure that the communication flow between the school and the *cottages* is unimpeded. One *girl's* reaction is:

> Even before I get back to the *cottage* the *staff* already knows how my day went. It makes me feel kind of important. Since the *memos* are coming anyway, I might as well try to make some good ones come my way. Also, the *staff* make a big fuss about them, write them down in my *log*. I tell my parents they can be proud of me when they come for family sessions.

The main part of the *team meeting* is taken up by planning the activities for the week and discussing short range treatment objectives for individual *girls.*

Team Requests

As Sally put it earlier, "the *team request* is quite an event around here." It is the encounter involving the largest number of participants, all the *team members* and all the *girls* in the group. The actors compare several readings of "how a *girl*'s week went." A *girl* presents her perception of her own performance, group members offer her feedback on how they saw her week from their different perspectives, and finally the *team members* voice their opinions, basing their observations on the various days of the week when they worked with her.

The *team request* is considered the climactic point of the week by all participants. During the first half of the week, expectations are built up in anticipation. Tuesday afternoon and Wednesday morning, staff members find the *girls* to be exceptionally good. Impression management, to use a Goffmanian phrase, is geared towards making sure they get their *team request.* The *docks,* or extra *charges* one gets for not completing regular *charges* properly, have to be worked off before one can ask for a *team request*.

During the second half of the week, "The *girls* act more in character," says the *cottage social worker* quoted earlier. He explains:

> Those who got their *team requests* have it "made." Now all they have to do is not cause any major blow-ups so they won't lose it. Those who didn't get it are mad and let you know it, as next week's *team request* is still far ahead.

He finds this to be a positive phenomenon:

> It gives them a concrete short-term goal to work for. If they can hold their act together for three days in a row, that's a good sign. You have something to build on.

Subgroups Within the Setting

Looking at various encounters that occur in the setting, one can distinguish several groups of actors with common goals, interests, or problems considered as sub-cultures in the present anthropological interpretation. Most actors belong to more than one such group. Some of the groups are created by the treatment philosophy itself, that is, that people with the same problems and interests constitute the best support system for each other. In accordance with this ideology, residents in a certain stage of the program can be regarded as a sub-culture, such as *new girls* or *girls on pre-release*.

There are also organizationally fostered sub-cultures among employees with similar roles and responsibilities, for example, the *cottage supervisors, cottage social workers,* and *night counselors.* While these are all horizontal sub-cultures, the cottage identity serves as a basis for a vertical sub-cultural affiliation as well, for both residents and staff members. It brings an element of challenge or competition into the system. The *girls* in school and in sports events express it in an attitude of "Our cottage is the best." They also bring back from these encounters an "It's done differently in that *cottage*" perspective. This makes for a constant re-evaluation of *cottage* routines and a readiness to try out new ways. Thus, the cultural identity of most actors is established through simultaneous membership in one or more vertical and one or more horizontal sub-cultures.

THE CENTER

Having looked at various parts of the setting, the actors, and the program, a picture of the *Center* gradually emerges. As I have already shown, conveying a sense of belonging to both residents and employees is a focal cultural value and a prerequisite for all other values to take hold. What are some of the ways in which this is achieved?

The *Springdale Weekly Bulletin,* which comes out on Wednesdays, keeps everybody abreast of the news, official and personal, happy and sad. Birthday cards, jubilee dinners in recognition of devoted service, Halloween parties, Thanksgiving and Christmas dinners for residents, employees, and their families, picnics, benefit concerts, and talent shows all contribute to creating a family atmosphere.

Many *former girls* look back on the period spent at Springdale as a most meaningful experience. Returning from an out-of-town trip to visit a *former girl* who had undergone surgery, the *program director* explains, "Several of them serve on our advisory board and many become involved in volunteer work years later."

EPILOGUE

I hope I have elucidated the metaphor of the treatment center as a cultural scene. If so, applying the anthropological perspective in the context of staff development and various education or training contexts may prove useful. Child care workers who realize that their organization is guided by a value system and has a language and a social structure of its own are better equipped to solve the overwhelmingly complex human problems they are facing daily.

Workers who are sensitized to the existence of differential interpretations of words, acts, and situations by various actors in their setting will be aware of the need to clarify meanings before taking action. This will result in improved communication, which makes for both better service to the client and better job satisfaction for the professional.

Chapter 3

Staff-Client Relations: A Critical Analysis

This chapter undertakes a critical analysis of staff-client relations. Youth care workers' and residents' behavior and attitudes towards manifestations of sick role behavior provide the context for this exploration. It starts out by considering a specific incident that can be regarded as a micro-cultural event, since it encapsulates overt and covert values as well as rules of conduct in the setting. This perspective helps workers better understand how and why such crisis situations can occur.

As a "mirror," this chapter documents staff dysfunctionality in handling crises and serves as an indictment of unprofessional practice. It marks the low ebb that staff-client relations can reach when workers act unreflectively and teams sink into an isolationist, the-world-as-the-cottage, stance.

The institution is the one to which we have been introduced in Chapter 2: An organization whose program was cohesive and values seemed clear. How could such deterioration set in? Our interest is not in the plot of the drama that occurred in a particular treatment center at a specific point in time. Rather, understanding the underlying conditions that might recur in other settings is what matters.

Chapter 2 dealt with socialization to overt values as made manifest in the program. Here dysfunctionality stems from unexamined practice and a lack of attention to the subtleties of the evolving

---

[Haworth co-indexing entry note]: "Staff-Client Relations: A Critical Analysis." Eisikovits, Rivka A. Co-published simultaneously in *Child & Youth Services* (The Haworth Press, Inc.) Vol. 18, No. 1, 1997, pp. 43-53; and: *The Anthropology of Child and Youth Care Work* (Rivka A. Eisikovits) The Haworth Press, Inc., 1997, pp. 43-53. Single or multiple copies of this article are available from The Haworth Document Delivery Service [1-800-342-9678, 9:00 a.m. - 5:00 p.m. (EST). E-mail address: getinfo@haworth.com].

cultural dynamics within the resident subsystem. Ongoing worker self-evaluation can prevent such crises.

In this worst-case scenario, workers relate to residents as if no program were in place and no individual treatment plans existed. They use "sick-role" language flippantly, without asking themselves where such terminology comes from and where it might lead. As demonstrated, it leads nowhere. It turns into a trap.

When one looks upon this selection as a "model," ways to avoid such dysfunctionality become apparent. The effectiveness of child and youth care workers depends on their ability to maintain ecologies that are congruent with the needs of society in order to prepare their charges to return as competent, functioning members. To achieve this, team coordination is crucial. Workers must continuously challenge one another's positions to prevent routinized action. Maintaining a holistic perspective on the cottage as part of a larger treatment organization and taking a longitudinal approach to residents' individual goals and needs, continuously reevaluating them in the light of client feedback, can serve as safety valves.

The value of a theoretical framework, the sick-role model (Parsons, 1957; Levine & Kozloff, 1978) in this case, to interpret behavior and to organize disparate pieces of interaction into a meaningful, albeit heuristic construct, is demonstrated. The careful, analogic application of a theoretical framework is shown to have both diagnostic and problem-solving potential.

The anthropologist's distancing technique–rendering the familiar strange and then familiar again–shows the way out of the impasse into which workers locked themselves due to over-involvement and loss of critical perspective.

No Exit: Residential Treatment and the "Sick-Role" Trap[1]

The idea that the medical model should be replaced by developmental educational models as the underlying philosophy of residen-

1. This selection is adapted from R. A. Eisikovits, "No Exit: Residential Treatment and the 'Sick Role' Trap," *Child Care Quarterly, 12*(1), 1983, with the permission of the editor and Human Sciences Press.

tial child care is by now widely accepted in the child care field (Eisikovits, Beker, & Guttmann, 1991; Maier, 1991; Whittaker, 1979). This is reflected in program descriptions in public relations brochures and in the expressions of program directors about their organizations' treatment philosophies. To assess its application in practice, however, one must also look at the programs themselves.

As an anthropologist doing fieldwork in a treatment center for delinquent girls, I had the chance to do both. The research findings indicate that while the professed treatment ideology endorses a developmental or educational approach to the residents, the treatment staff tend to view their clients as if they were "sick," based on the mere fact of their placement in a residential setting. Argyris and Schon (1974) refer to these as "espoused theory" and "theory-in-use" respectively. The basic discrepancy between these two philosophies, and the staff's unawareness of using them selectively in spite of their contradictory nature, explains many of the frequent communication failures between staff and residents.

In view of this finding, Parsons' (1957, p. 440) sick-role model appeared to be a rewarding framework for understanding the staff-client interactions. Its main tenets are that:

1. the person in the sick role is exempted from normal social responsibilities;
2. depending on the nature and severity of the illness, it is understood that he or she is in need of care and cannot recover without professional help;
3. although one is not "blamed" for one's condition, the sick person must define his or her state as undesirable; and
4. he or she has to comply with the instructions of the professional, usually a physician, who charts the course of recovery and is, in fact, the legitimizer of the sick role.

Despite the impressive volume of social science literature on the subject, some of it critical, Parsons' formulation has determined the course of research on the topic (Levine & Kozloff, 1978).

The pattern tends to be highlighted when someone in the cottage "really" gets sick, thus upsetting the equilibrium of the system. The following field note excerpt is illustrative:

> On my way to the cottage I heard a chorus of shrill agitated voices shouting, "Get her out of here!" "Take her to the hospital where she belongs!" "Why are you all fussing around her?" I soon learned that the reason for the turmoil was Sandy, a sixteen-year-old diabetic who had a severe attack the day before her release was scheduled.

Following the assumption that the institution can be regarded as a cultural system with its own language, values, rules of proper conduct, and social structure, as we have seen in Chapter 2, this incident can be considered as a "micro-cultural event." Any interaction in which participants act in accordance with cultural norms can be so designated and used as a basis for understanding the cultural system within which it occurred (Burnett, 1973).

If one examines the girls' reactions to Sandy's diabetic attack in this light, the essence of their concerns emerges:

1. to remove her because her presence constitutes a threat: "Get her out of here !"
2. to place her in the proper settings for persons in her condition: "Take her to the hospital where she belongs."

The implication is that she violates a cultural norm by her very presence in the setting. She usurps a role or status which is not judged to be rightfully hers by the rest of the residents, thus evoking feelings of jealousy and attempts to restore the upset equilibrium: "Why are you all fussing around her?" Even stronger is the girls' unexpressed but implied reproach: ". .. instead of fussing around us," which brings the episode to a climax.

Having to deal with a chronically ill girl distracted the staff's attention from the other residents–her acute condition seemed to justify her being "fussed about." The importance of being "fussed about" is a commonly shared value linked to the sick-role that regulates staff-client interaction, to be referred to later as the "attention giving and seeking" interaction compound.

Thus the girl's urgent need competed with and tended to invalidate the legitimacy of their claims to the privileges of the sick-role: (1) exemption from normal responsibilities and (2) a recognition of their need for special attention and their inability to recover on their own. The study found that the manifestations of both physical and psychosomatic illness within the institution become classified by the residents according to a single criterion: Does it enhance or diminish the claimant's chances to achieve sick-role status?

The idea will be developed through an exploration of what the residents and the staff classify as legitimate and illegitimate sick-roles in the institution, demonstrating the consensus that residency is the only legitimate basis for claiming sick-role privileges over an extended period. Attention-giving and attention-seeking will be viewed as fundamental to the interaction between staff and the legitimate sick-role incumbents. It will be shown how and why the sick-role model becomes dysfunctional and leads to an impasse in the treatment process.

RESIDENTS' ATTITUDES TO PHYSICAL AND MENTAL ILLNESS

The girls' attitudes toward physical illness vary according to the severity of the condition. Acute cases are perceived as a threat to the healthy residents' claim to sick-role status, but minor ailments that do not draw too much attention from others in the group are accepted. They help dramatize the resident's claim for attention and exemption from regular duties. Arriving at the cottage, I would often be greeted by girls with the latest news: "You know, I had the flu!" or, "I had an infection so I'm still on antibiotics. Don't forget to get me my medicine!"

Being diagnosed as mentally ill or retarded is seen as a real danger in the resident sub-culture. It is interpreted to mean that the staff consider the person to be a hopeless case and may even cause one to be transferred to a psychiatric ward. Therefore, manifestations of psychosomatic or mental disorder lead to rejection and are dreaded (Reiter & Bryen, 1991), as shown in the following illustrations:

> Linda, a 15 year old epileptic, used this cultural knowledge to frighten her peers. She bragged about her palm reading ability and claimed to "hear voices," so the girls associated her illness with occult forces and excluded her from most of their activities. The counselors interpreted her behavior as revenge

> for being shunned by the rest of the girls in the cottage for "having fits."
>
> Lisa, 14, whose mother was mentally retarded, was embarrassed whenever her mother talked to a staff member on the phone. She once burst out in a group meeting: "You all look at me like I was mental just 'cause my Mom is." She could only sleep with the lights on and had recurring nightmares but refused to see the institution's psychologist because "I won't let any shrink mess my head up."

So far it has been demonstrated that the girls' attitudes to various manifestations of illness is generally negative. However, one version of the sick-role unanimously considered desirable is to be diagnosed as chemically dependent. This grants privileges that enhance the role incumbent's prestige, e.g., the chemically dependent resident can leave the premises. "Now I get to go to Team House for AA meetings and I can always meet cute guys there."

Several attributes of this type of sick-role make it attractive for the girls. The first of the Twelve Steps, the Alcoholics Anonymous (1952) philosophy adhered to in the institution, calls upon the addict to admit his or her helplessness in controlling substance-related behavior, hence allowing a passive stance, at least at the beginning. It requires little effort and it is a sure attention-getter from both staff and parents: "Now, at least my folks have to realize they better take me seriously."

The greatest advantage of the chemically dependent status is that it is a permanent sick role. AA members are encouraged to perceive themselves as chemically dependent for the rest of their lives, which means the sick role need not be cast off. It can be safely taken along upon leaving the institution and integrated into one's permanent social identity (Goodenough, 1966, p. 181). Some of the skills the AA member has acquired also prove to be usable in various other self-help groups, thereby enhancing the role incumbent's social standing. If one were to place the residents' attitudes toward various illness manifestations on a scale, mental or psychosomatic conditions would appear at the negative end and chemical dependency would constitute the positive extreme.

Youth counselors usually treat instances of physical illness as "con-jobs" or "cop-outs from duty." They hesitate to hand out even the most common pain reliever when a girl first complains about some physical discomfort, preferring to wait to see whether the symptom will intensify. Their suspiciousness is not without foundation, since the girls often feign or exaggerate their symptoms, but this, in turn, leads the girls to put on a more convincing show.

Such situations can become dangerous when acute conditions are involved. A striking example was the reaction of one youth counselor who slept in the cottage the night of Sandy's diabetic attack. "I have seen her work herself up to this state before," the worker said when she saw Sandy vomiting and hyperventilating. "She wants to avoid facing the reality of leaving." Thus, the counselor applied the "con-job" approach at a stage of the illness when the girl was no longer able to control her condition. By the time she was taken to the hospital, Sandy was in a diabetic coma. In other words, the staff also tend to play down manifestations of physical illness, mostly treating them as setting-inappropriate behaviors. They, too, consider residency as the only "legitimate" basis for sick-role status in the institution.

ATTENTION GIVING AND SEEKING

The need of the residents for care is implicitly recognized by the staff, who translate their own complementary role into behavioral terms as attention-giving. The log serves to remind staff members to spend time daily with each resident, dispensing attention in individual and in group sessions.

Each girl's day in school is also carefully arranged to assure opportunities for proper allocation of attention. In the small school located on campus and offering a special education program, the girls attend classes in groups of up to eight students, permitting individualized instructional techniques to be employed. An intricate communication network is set up to acknowledge both positive and negative behavior in school. The teacher who serves as a liaison between the two subsystems, school and cottage, briefs her colleagues every morning on meaningful events in the girls' lives. "Betty had a haircut, be sure to notice it!"; "Yesterday was Sue's shopping day; remember to compliment her on her new outfit."

Unaware of the fact that they are the ones responsible for organizing the day around attention-giving, the staff relate to girls' attention-seeking behaviors as if they were diagnostic indicators. Instead of addressing the real problems that brought the clients to the institution, they end up using girls' style of socialization to the resident role as a basis for their individual treatment plans. This application of the sick-role model converts the setting into a total institution and reflects the distinction made by Seidl (1974) between mediatory and total institutions according to the goal of treatment. In the first type, the institution serves as a vehicle for enhancing the client's community readjustment, whereas in the second, the adjustment to the institutional setting becomes the main objective.

"Classical rebel" is the label staff attach to those residents who refuse to assume the ready-made cultural identity provided by the sick role smoothly and insist on playing the game according to their own rules instead, at least at the beginning. Behaviors characteristic of this category include attempts to run away while making sure one is caught, "bitching" when a youth counselor is within hearing distance, dressing inappropriately for various occasions such as wearing a long skirt for school, or donning insufficient clothing in cold weather "'cause only softies put on a dozen tops." Many of these behavioral patterns revolve around clothing and makeup as the most obvious vehicles for presentation of self (Goffman, 1959).

"Honeymooners," on the other hand, are those girls who willingly assume the sick-role: they readily "share feelings in group," ask for "group time and staff support" to cope with their problems, and "do their charges." Why the staff dislike the "rebels" is obvious, but it seems that the "honeymooners" constitute a suspect group, too. The assumption that the "honeymooners" merely "front" compliance is inherent in the label. The following remarks are indicative: "She can probably hold it together for a few more days," or "I wonder when she will show us her teeth." All the girls are placed along the "honeymooner"–"classical rebel" continuum. Rather than working on their individual problems at their own pace, they learn to adjust to these unwritten rules or expectations.

Staff members' frequent use of theater jargon suggests their awareness of the girls' role behavior, e.g., "Susan acted out of character." They also classify and interpret residents' behavior according to where in the cottage it took place. They call the downstairs area, where the girls may want to impress the staff, "the forestage." The upstairs, where the girls can "sometimes just be without any mask," as one youth counselor put it, is called, accordingly, "backstage."

The inconsistencies in the youth counselors' attitudes are evident. At the same time that they expect behavior changes, they also reproach the girls for "creaking performances" or dismiss their positive behavior as "mere play-acting." They appear to be either unaware of their own role as directors of the overall production or incapable of doing much about it.

WHEN THE "SICK-ROLE" CRACKS AND CRUMBLES

According to the Parsonian model (Parsons, 1957), the sick role is a transient one which the patient first assumes, then discards upon recovery. As interpreted in this institution, however, though helpful in daily living, the sick-role becomes equated with institutional life. Thus, it fails to provide any guidance to the residents struggling to find their way out of either the role or the institution. Instead, it becomes permanent and dysfunctional, thus reinforcing those organizational patterns that serve to make adjustment to the institution the primary goal.

On the level of its professed treatment philosophy, the institution provides each resident with an individual treatment plan. However, the implementation of these plans becomes problematic for several reasons. The logistics of memorizing and operationalizing each resident's treatment goals seem hard to manage in a cottage housing twelve girls, with two youth counselors on duty who have many additional responsibilities.

An even more substantial reason for not applying the individual treatment plans that are part of a complex developmental model is the counselors' lack of adequate training. The medical approach, on the other hand, offers a more immediately tangible task for the youth-counselor-turned-therapist, at least in the short run. The needs of the resident-as-patient are immediate. Providing attention becomes the equivalent of handing out a pain reliever and carries a sense of relative fulfillment: "I have done something real for her today."

The girls, for their part, with the exception of the "classical rebels," had initially assumed the sick-role because of its short-range advantages. But they find themselves at an impasse when they wish to discard the sick-role and exhibit "healthy" behavior instead, in order to be released. "But all I have learned here is how to bitch" is a typical resident complaint. The girls do not feel that they have learned any systematic skills that help them demonstrate behavioral changes that would lead to their discharge.

At this point, since the staff cannot provide specific guidelines to assist them, the girls are referred to the professed treatment modality, i.e., the developmental model, which is present in the description of the program but not in the operational treatment process. Despite structural provisions such as periodic treatment plan reviews and program labels for the various stages of the institutional experience, there are no behaviorally specific criteria spelled out for the girls to follow.

It is no wonder that the girls, intolerant of such ambiguity, turn the tables and accuse the staff of using a "con-job" approach. Many have had prior institutional experiences in custodially oriented settings in which the expectations were clearer. The physical attractiveness of the setting, home-like decoration, extensive grounds, and lack of lockups only serve to confuse them, and they conclude that these are nothing more than a deceptive facade.

When they hear the youth counselors announce: "We don't force anyone to stay here, girls have to choose to stay," their standard reactions are: "Are you saying that you're giving me permission to go?" or, "Man, I would leave any moment!" One girl expressed her feeling most vividly by asking: "Why should lions pretend to be lambs? To me they're lions no matter what!"

Even though the youth counselors are unable to pronounce their "patients" cured on the basis of any inherent professional criteria, residence has to be terminated at some point. External variables, such as the refusal of many counties to pay beyond a certain period or the advent of a "timely" court hearing, often intervene to rescue staff and residents alike from the dead end to which the application of an unsuitable treatment model has led them.

CONCLUSIONS

Although the forgoing analysis is based on staff-client interactions observed in a particular institution, the kinds of problems highlighted stem from shortcomings that other such settings are likely to share. Discrepancies of this kind between espoused theories and theories-in-use, more often vaguely sensed than actually demonstrated in residential care, may result in the immobilization of an entire program. Not only are clients not properly or effectively served, but the reputation of the organization is harmed, as well. Child care workers end up trapped in a vicious cycle. They become frustrated and soon "burn out." The need for careful examination of the correspondence between what we do and what we think we do with youngsters in institutions emerges forcefully in this context.

Chapter 4

A Comparative Study of Subsystem Relations in Two Child and Youth Care Organizations

In the following selection the relationship between the treatment and education subsystems in two child and youth care organizations, referred to as Springdale and Autumnville, is compared. Variance in this relationship produces discrepant client experiences and yields different results.

A holistic ethnographic picture of the Springdale residential setting has been provided in Chapter 2, on the basis of which we can proceed to a more focused study of issues and relationships. Nevertheless, as Chapter 3 has made clear, the cultures of such settings cannot be assumed to be immutable. They are in constant flux, and effective work depends on taking these shifts into account.

Since Springdale is the setting the reader has come to know quite intimately from the previous two chapters, it is used here as the basis for the inter-organizational comparison. This does not mean, however, that parameters derived from one context are arbitrarily applied in the analysis of the other. Autumnville must also be presented in sufficient detail to come alive. Although Springdale has been described in Chapter 2, relevant parts of the description are brought here again to allow a balanced and meaningful comparison.

[Haworth co-indexing entry note]: "A Comparative Study of Subsystem Relations in Two Child and Youth Care Organizations." Eisikovits, Rivka A. Co-published simultaneously in *Child & Youth Services* (The Haworth Press, Inc.) Vol. 18, No. 1, 1997, pp. 55-65; and: *The Anthropology of Child and Youth Care Work* (Rivka A. Eisikovits) The Haworth Press, Inc., 1997, pp. 55-65. Single or multiple copies of this article are available from The Haworth Document Delivery Service [1-800-342-9678, 9:00 a.m. - 5:00 p.m. (EST). E-mail address: getinfo@haworth.com].

Just as one can pick up crucial information about the setting from a micro-cultural incident, so too can a routine daily event, like the group conversation around the kitchen table, reveal significant features of the local culture. At Springdale, girls share their feelings and experiences freely, so the youth counselor plays a relatively passive role, listening and reinforcing them when needed (see page 57). At Autumnville during the dialogue between the resident and the researcher (see page 58), the latter asks open-ended questions influencing the interviewee only minimally. In both of these cases the adult participants do not determine the course of interaction. In other instances, however, child and youth care workers might take a more directive stance. For a contextual analysis of clients' actions or responses, practitioners have to consider their own input into the situation under study.

To gain a holistic view of the role of the school, a number of sources are tapped: clients' perspectives are sought; official descriptions of the programs as they appear in orientation packages for new staff are consulted; and the role of the school as perceived by treatment and school personnel is included as well. If differences of opinion exist, this approach brings them to the surface. The inquiry proceeds from specific viewpoints to the larger context of ideas, leading to the formulation of a heuristic model of optimal relations between the treatment and educational subsystems in child and youth care organizations.

Detotalizing the Institutional Experience: The Role of the School in the Residential Treatment of Juveniles[1]

SCENARIO I–SPRINGDALE

[It is 2:30 pm, and the girls are sitting around a dining room table in the cottage, drinking hot chocolate and discussing their day in school with Diane, one of their youth counselors.]

---

1. This selection is adapted from R. A. Eisikovits & Z. Eisikovits, "Detotalizing the Institutional Experience: The Role of the School in the Residential Treatment of Juveniles," *Residential & Community Child Care Administration*, 1(4), 1980, with the permission of the second author.

Grace: I had a super day in school today. Mrs. Brown [the Home Economics teacher] said my pea soup was the highlight of the mini-restaurant! Danny was there and some of the other social workers came for lunch, and I got lots of compliments from everybody.

Diane: Yay for Grace!!!

Judy: I had an ok day too. I guess a memo is coming telling you guys [this was directed to the youth counselor] about it. Mrs. West says I'm reading at my grade level now. I could hardly believe it. Wait 'til my Mom finds out! At my old school they used to say I was too far behind to catch up.

Pat: I started working on a new piece for the guitar. The talent show is in two weeks, you know.

Laurie: Mrs. Bright said we really have a good softball team this year. Guess what she told me. She said I was one of the key players!

Diane: That's wonderful, Laurie.

Arlene [a new girl]: You seem to be doing different things in school than I am.

Judy: That's because we are in all different classes.

Arlene: Sounds like it gives you stuff to talk about in the cottage. Not like when you all go to the same classes. That bores me to death.

Grace: This way it's easier to make more friends. You get close with girls from other cottages.

Arlene: I get you. When they jump on your case in the cottage you've still got someone to talk to.

Diane: Real good observation, Arlene.

SCENARIO II–AUTUMNVILLE

[In the cottage in the afternoon]

Researcher: Can you talk about school?

Resident [a 16 year old Caucasian male]: On the outs or in here?

Researcher: In here.

Resident: Well, school is just another thing we do with the group. They say all kids have to do some school work. So they figure out what are the things you can carry and what you have to learn and they fit you in some program. But you go with your group. In a way it's nicer than on the outs. You go slower and stuff . . .

Researcher: How about the teachers?

Resident: Like any place. Some are nice, some sticky . . . They fill in your group leader about how you are doing in school, everyday, the dudes, too . . . They bring up in group shit you've been doing in school. Like if you show a problem, get small feelings or something they'd know it right away.

Researcher: That's interesting. Tell me more about it.

Resident: Like, you know, dudes in my cottage know a lot about my shit. They know when I get aggravated and when I'm pissed I don't really care about nothin'. So when things get messy in school they kinda mess it up for you all the way.

These are two excerpts from the field notes: the "highlight of the day" for the former, "just another thing we do" for the latter. What makes the educational experience in the juvenile institution a worthwhile one from the residents' perspective? What are the possible organizational gains from taking the clients' perspective into account? For a complete "insider" picture to emerge, it is necessary to allow the actors in the social system under study to speak for themselves.

The clients' perspective (scenarios) is followed by official descriptions of the two programs as they appear in orientation material packages for new staff. Then the role of the school, as perceived by both treatment and school personnel, is presented. Subsequently a comparative analysis of the cultural context of the treatment programs and their underlying philosophies is undertaken to provide a basis for understanding the variance in the residents' schooling experience. Finally, a heuristic model is proposed that will optimize the relationship between the treatment and educational components of residential programs for adolescents to enhance durable change.

THE RESEARCH SITES

Two residential treatment facilities were studied: one for girls; the other, co-educational but housing a predominantly male population. The former, Springdale, is a private, non-profit organization with a capacity of 55 residents. The client population is composed of adolescent girls aged 14-18 with a range of emotional, behavioral, and social adjustment problems. They are referred through the Juvenile Courts and various other social service agencies.

Springdale is located in the suburbs of a moderately large city and has a private lake and a variety of indoor and outdoor recreational facilities. Each of the girls lives in a separate room in one of five cottages, which are designed and decorated to create a homelike atmosphere. A public school offering a special education program is located on campus. The school is meant to serve day students from the surrounding community as well as the residents. All of the facilities are modern.

The second research site, here called Autumnville, is a state-operated juvenile institution with a capacity of 150 residents. One cottage, populated by females, is not included in the study population. All youth here have been committed to the State Department of Corrections.

Autumnville is located in a small town. The large campus includes eight cottages, an administration building, a chapel, a dining room, a variety of shops, and a school. Some of the buildings are more than one hundred years old; the others have been built recently. The meticulously kept grounds and freshly painted buildings create a somewhat sterile atmosphere. The cottages are clean and uniformly furnished and decorated. The number of residents per room varies according to room size, and considerations of treatment and control. The school is located in a separate building and has a special program of remedial learning. It serves only the residents.

TREATMENT PHILOSOPHY AND PROGRAM

Orientation packages for new staff, used as a medium of socialization, constitute a reliable source for understanding an organization's manifest ideology. The following excerpts from these materials are illustrative:

> *Springdale*: . . . The overall philosophy of treatment is based on the concept that treatment deals with the total person . . . Staff must bow before the mystery of each person and accept the limitations to understanding her . . . Behavior is only an outward manifestation of a person . . . Staff will look beyond the behavior in evaluating and responding to it in practice . . . Since the girl is capable of change but cannot be coerced she is ultimately responsible for her own behavior.

The above major tenets of treatment philosophy shape the treatment program, which is individualized and includes a considerable degree of flexibility. Following a three-week period of diagnosis and adjustment, a treatment plan is drawn up for each resident with her active participation.

Role modeling and providing a therapeutic milieu are two of the core values introduced in both individual and group counseling situations. Staff are given considerable latitude to interpret the treatment philosophy and are expected to develop "a personal way of expressing care and love."

At Autumnville, on the other hand, Positive Peer Culture (PPC) (Vorrath & Brendtro, 1974) constitutes the philosophical base of the program, as reflected in the institution's training manual:

> *Autumnville*: . . . Youth are delinquent primarily because of their poor relationships with other people, poor self-concepts, and their past inability to handle themselves responsibly . . . Youth are profoundly influenced by associations with their peers . . . PPC is designed to turn around a negative youth subculture and mobilize the power of the peer group in a productive manner.

In PPC, youths assume the task of giving help rather than getting help. In line with the above philosophy the major treatment device in the institution is the group. All daily activities are structured around it. The focus of the group process is on the existential present as reflected in the members' everyday life rather than on deep-seated, past-related problems. Youths are socialized to put their problems in clear, behaviorally specific language and to fit them into one of nine areas believed to encompass the full range of possible behavioral problems. Each has a specific name: easily misled or misleads others, light fingering, lying, drinking . . . , inconsiderate, fronting, easily aggravated, and small feelings.

Three major concepts are at the heart of this philosophy: The power of the peer group, the importance of giving help instead of getting help, and the role of those already "reformed" in understanding and reforming peers with problems similar to their own.

PERSPECTIVES ON THE ROLE OF THE SCHOOL

Springdale. Views on the role of the school in this institution vary. The program director perceives it as an integral part of the treatment program; therefore, the school principal appears on the organizational chart of the treatment center as reporting to the program director.

From interviewing the principal, however, a different perspective emerges. The latter emphasizes the autonomous character of the school. He dwells on points of divergence between the manifest ideologies of the two organizations, speaking extensively about services rendered to the community and the day students to highlight the school's public character. He also brings up the issue of the school's image in the community resulting from its location in a juvenile treatment center.

Nevertheless, he describes the relations between the institution and the school as based on mutuality and exchange of services. For example, the institution provides the facilities and the public school district pays the teachers' salaries. The importance of efficient collaboration in the best interest of the clients/students is recognized unanimously.

Accordingly, a representative of the school participates in intake interviews to help map out school-related problems and potential solutions on the initial treatment plan. The principal interviews every candidate and takes an active part in the decision to accept a new resident based on educational considerations such as projected ability to benefit from an individualized educational program, carry responsibility, etc. A holistic, individualized approach to clients/students provides the ideological grounds for this cooperation.

Autumnville. The superintendent as well as the treatment director perceive schooling as an organic part of the treatment sequence. School difficulties are regarded as symptomatic of the general problems faced by the youth. Thus, the school personnel are not only involved but submerged in the treatment process. They, too, see the school as a diagnostic and treatment tool. While working on his "problem areas," the resident also takes care of his educational needs.

Reflecting the marginal or subsidiary role of the school in the institution, the organizational chart identifies the school principal as an "education coordinator." Illustrative of the same point is the fact that, although a student can get academic credit for fulfilling school requirements, high school graduation is available only through GED tests or outside community schools that agree to award diplomas to those who have fulfilled requirements equivalent to theirs.

COMPARATIVE ANALYSIS

Comparing the two treatment philosophies, one realizes that the term "philosophy" itself is used differently in the two settings. At Springdale it stands for a moral philosophy assuming a holistic view of man, whereas at Autumnville it is used to refer to the program. Having made this distinction, the term will be used as an insiders' category in continuation.

There is a conceptual divergence on the anatomy of change as well. At Springdale, change is regarded as an act of individual choice. The program is process-oriented and is pursued on the basis of individual treatment plans. At Autumnville, change is viewed as generally occurring only under pressure. By intent, the individual's freedom of choice is limited. The program is goal-oriented, designed to achieve changed behavior patterns in pre-determined areas. Being constantly confronted by his peers, the client experiences change as agony rather than as growth.

In line with the holistic approach adopted at Springdale, the client is seen as part of her family; hence her problems are interpreted on the level of family system problems. This means that she is seen as only partially responsible for her situation. At Autumnville, on the other hand, the client is expected and pressured to take full responsibility for his existential situation and not use family problems as "excuses" or "leaning posts." Home visits at Springdale are regarded as part of the program, as they offer residents the opportunity to practice new learning under natural conditions. At Autumnville, on the other hand, the home visit is viewed as extraneous to the program, a privilege to be earned. This means that the communication or problem solving skills the youth acquires in the institution may rarely, if ever, be tried out beyond the PPC group.

The variance in the degree of family involvement in the programs is reflected in societal attitudes towards the institutions and perceptions of the kinds of learning that occur within them. The competencies acquired at Springdale are often appreciated by the resident's family. It is not uncommon for the client to become a change agent in her own family, taking the position of moderator in decision making and role-setting processes.

The minimal family involvement at Autumnville reduces the visibility of learning that occurs in the institution. The client is looked upon as the black sheep of the family, and the institution as a place where errant youths are supposed to straighten out. Hence there is little recognition of knowledge acquired in the institution as applicable outside, and no status change in the family accompanies the client's successful completion of the program.

Positive experiences lead to the internalization of the value of change and of improved communication at Springdale. Moreover, the ability to transfer relational skills outside the institution is a major yardstick for successful completion of the program.

At Autumnville, on the other hand, where youth maintain simultaneous membership in two distinct cultural systems, that of the program and that of the peers, internalization of values in general and of change in particular is almost impossible. By denying the existence of a "backstage" where the norms of the delinquent subculture prevail, the treatment staff defeats the main goal of the program, i.e., "turning around the delinquent peer culture into a positive peer culture." Without such internalization, no individual or cultural system can be durably changed.

CONCLUSIONS

From the foregoing comparative analysis and from matching the perceptions of treatment personnel, school administration, and clients concerning the place of the school, some inferences can be drawn regarding the quality of the educational experience in the institutions and the relationship between that and the organization's treatment goals.

When the school is organizationally perceived by both treatment and school personnel as an integral part of an overall treatment program and the educational model is subordinated to the treatment model, the client's educational experience cannot serve as a guide for lasting change. The treatment/medical model is geared for "curing" and does not recognize the need to perpetuate change once the client is pronounced cured and leaves the institution. This makes going to school just "another thing we do." When the members of the treatment group and the school group are identical, the unchanging audience witnessing the total range of the individual's daily activities has a totalizing effect (Goffman, 1961) on the institutional experience. The centrality of school in the youth's life outside the institution is in no way reflected in the subordinated role of the school within the institution.

When, on the other hand, the school within the institution operates according to an educational philosophy of its own, the educational model complements the treatment goals of the program. Aiming to effect lasting change, it helps the client internalize this value.

When the residents are allowed to put together their school programs, thereby introducing an important element of individual choice into the system, the treatment and school groups are no longer identical. Changes occur in both adult and peer audiences—teachers vs. treatment personnel (social workers, youth counselors), and schoolmates vs. the cottage group. Thus the school has a detotalizing effect on the individual's institutional experience. It provides opportunities for trying out various roles and for practicing newly acquired relational skills.

The practical implications of the organizational alternatives described above are significant. They point not only to the way in which the school can have a major detotalizing effect on the residents' institutional experience, but also illuminate the need to allow subsystems within the institution a considerable degree of autonomy to relate to residents according to criteria flowing out of their professional ideologies, e.g., as clients in treatment, as students in school, as players in sports and other recreational activities. Such a policy provides an organizational safety valve against client stereotyping, helps to normalize the clients' experiences, creates the conditions for producing lasting change, and paves the road back to the community.

Chapter 5

Cultural and Futures Perspectives on the Residential Education Alternative

The previous chapter looked at interaction modalities between organizational subsystems and their effects on clients' experience and program outcomes. This one takes a broad perspective on the institution-society nexus, viewing residential settings as adaptive mechanisms within a macro-culture's ecology.

It has three parts. The first analyzes changing trends in the use of residential arrangements within one national-cultural context to map out conditions under which they served social needs optimally. The following two parts attempt to identify how these environments could be employed in the future for both normative student populations and those who require residential services for special problems.

As is demonstrated in Chapter 1, exposure to the anthropological model can enable child and youth care workers to become flexible and versatile facilitators of cultural learning. These qualities enhance their effectiveness as leaders in such innovative programs.

Jesco von Puttkamer (1983), a noted NASA programs analyst, argues that humanity's peak accomplishments in such key areas as transportation, energy, food production, and health care were all made possible by holistic thinking. Jesuit paleontologist and philosopher Teilhard de Chardin (1965) argues that progress in the social domain parallel to these unprecedented leaps in the technological

---

[Haworth co-indexing entry note]: "Cultural and Futures Perspectives on the Residential Education Alternative." Eisikovits, Rivka A. Co-published simultaneously in *Child & Youth Services* (The Haworth Press, Inc.) Vol. 18, No. 1, 1997, pp. 67-78; and: *The Anthropology of Child and Youth Care Work* (Rivka A. Eisikovits) The Haworth Press, Inc., 1997, pp. 67-78. Single or multiple copies of this article are available from The Haworth Document Delivery Service [1-800-342-9678, 9:00 a.m. - 5:00 p.m. (EST). E-mail address: getinfo@haworth.com].

sphere is hampered because fragmentation dominates the major paradigms of thinking of those involved.

Analyzing the functions that child and youth care institutions have fulfilled in various historic-cultural environments helps us to better grasp emerging directions in the field. Understanding the conditions under which maximal suitability to societal and individual needs has been attained is a precondition for effective planning. This chapter examines the roles of residential settings from three different angles. It starts out with a longitudinal investigation of their utilization in the Israeli sociocultural context, then proceeds to explore the future potential of the residential educational alternative for youth in general.

Finally, it takes a heuristic look at possible changes in this service delivery modality for "traditional" residential clients.

A.
Residential Education and Care in Cultural Context: An Israeli Example[1]

Comparatively studying the relationship between political systems and schools in various societies, anthropologist Yehudi Cohen (1975) writes:

> The analysis of the development of specific social institutions depends on the premise that social forms can only emerge, flourish, and be sustained in sociocultural atmospheres that are conducive to them. Each of these social forms must be regarded as an aspect of a population's adaptation to its total environment. (p. 103)

The use to which a society puts its institutions for children and youth is a good measure of its long range goals. Israel is a suitable context for analyzing the social functions of children's institutions

1. This selection is adapted from R. A. Eisikovits, "Children's Institutions in Israel as Mirrors of Social and Cultural Change," *Child & Youth Services, 7*(3/4), 1985.

from this perspective. Close to 20% of the nation's youth are educated in residential settings (Kashti, Arieli, & Wozner, 1981).

Cohen (1975) also maintains that, while:

> Man may affect the character of the institutions he creates, their emergence in the first place, or their loss, are not matters of deliberate social policy. (p. 109)

However, if their "character" at any given time is out of touch with the needs of society, this can bring about their "loss." A less deterministic stance than the one put forth by Cohen, the latter is a proposition against which the changing roles of residential education in Israel can be fruitfully assessed.

Day schools in most western democracies define their purpose as primarily one of training the mind and teaching subject matter; they are only minimally preoccupied with moral or ideological training. It is assumed that in the more comprehensive and supervised residential environment, a more holistic educational experience can be provided. This educational alternative can be considered to have advantages over day schooling if one or several of the following objectives prevail:

1. When character formation is the aim of formal education.
2. When the need for a total and supervised ideological immersion of the young is of primary national interest.
3. When education for membership in a social elite is the goal.

In his classic study of the role of schools in revolutionary, conservative, and reactionary societies, Wallace (1961) compares the relative position of primary and secondary socializing agencies under such political regimes. In revolutionary societies, he contends, the state claims close to complete control over the whole child at the expense of the family. The family's child-caring mandate is minimized because it is considered a subversive institution. This makes residential education a favored option.

In the former U.S.S.R., particularly in its earlier days, a high percentage of children were educated in boarding schools (Bronfenbrenner, 1970; Pearson, 1990). During the pre-statehood period in Israel, a highly idealistic orientation combined with the consequences of the Holocaust, which left many orphans in need of care (Wolins, 1971), made residential schools a socially adaptive alternative. In the United States, on the other hand, where individualism and self-determination have traditionally been focal values (Bellah et al., 1985; Wolins, 1974, p. 289), boarding schools tended to be viewed as more appropriate for "problematic" than for normal children.[1]

The essence of schooling, according to Cohen (1975), is to promote the adoption of universalistic criteria and standards of performance. Using the example of residential education in Israel, it is here demonstrated that only as long as a congruity between universalistic and particularistic or sectorial values prevails can coherence between educational goals and means be maintained.

The Pre-Statehood Period

Residential schools existed ever since the beginning of the Zionist settlement.[2] Some functioned as an integral part of various kibbutzim. Others were operated as organizationally autonomous entities, such as the agricultural boarding schools or youth villages that attempted to recreate and instill in their students the pioneering spirit that the kibbutz came to symbolize (Kashti, 1993).

These schools served several categories of students: the offspring of rural Jewish settlers and urban Zionists, new immigrant youth who had received a preparatory Zionist and agricultural education in their countries of origin prior to their arrival, and refugee children from the Nazi Holocaust who were brought to Israel by Youth Aliyah to start a new life (Kashti, Arieli, & Wozner, 1981). With a correspondence between universalistic and particularistic educational goals in place, residential schools proved to be optimally suited to societal needs. Talking about educating Youth Aliyah's charges, Wolins (1971) has put this most succinctly:

> Absorption meant preparation for membership in a kibbutz and for citizenship in the country. It meant the acceptance of an egalitarian, collectivist ideology, a life of labor on the land, self-fulfillment through group and even national accomplishment. (p. 5)

The Post-Statehood Scene

After the establishment of the state, this balance was gradually upset. The breaking point occurred with the founding of a state-supported educational system providing universal free schooling. Revolutionary pioneering zeal gave way to a more "established" social climate. In line with Wallace's (1961) theory, the importance of schools as central socializing agents declined with the advent of a more conservative stage in the political sphere. Families and communities came to be regarded as "trustworthy" primary socializers and residential schools lost their edge.

A rapid trend towards urbanization took place in the 1950s, and with it came a shift in value orientation from egalitarianism to individualism (Eisenstadt, 1973; Elboim-Dror, 1989). In an increasingly meritocratic system, credentials became the vehicles for upward mobility. Following independence, the absorption of immigrants was considered to be primarily the concern of the state. Immigrants' commitment to Zionist ideology could not be taken for granted. Those from Arab countries fled from persecution following Israel's independence, whereas European Jews, shattered by the Nazi Holocaust, brought along a more pragmatic orientation. The ineffectiveness of the kibbutz-based residential schools in absorbing these postwar immigrant children, most of whom arrived with their families rather than alone, became apparent.

Residential education was formally divorced from the increasingly particularistic ideological climate of the kibbutz and became an institutionalized branch of the national educational system, with Youth Aliyah as an ongoing partner. Nevertheless, it continued to promote an anachronistic, romanticized view of agrarianism because of its perceived inherent character-building value. At the same time in the rapidly changing, technologically oriented urban context, specialized education gained ascendancy, replacing the previously held ideal of a universal curriculum (Wolins, 1971).

During the first two decades of statehood, the provision of equal educational opportunity became a paramount issue for this ethnically heterogeneous society, absorbing massive immigration from East and West. The melting pot approach encouraged a differential pace of acculturation for representatives of the various generations within the immigrant family (Frankenstein, 1951). The placement of talented youngsters into residential schools appeared promising based on the assumption that there they could be socialized to the new norms more effectively (Frankenstein, 1961; Rottenschtreich, 1951).

No longer called upon to fulfill an *in loco parentis* role, many residential schools nevertheless continued to perceive socialization and character formation as their primary educational objective. Although most programs had added a vocational education component, it was generally considered by the staff to be of minor importance (Smilansky, Kashti, & Arieli, 1982). On the other hand, the students and their parents, predominantly of Sephardi (Asian and African) origin, were primarily interested in these vocational or career-oriented components, which they viewed as their chance for upward mobility. This goal ambiguity eroded parental support for residential schooling.

Due to the inter-ethnic and inter-generational tensions it produced, the melting pot model of absorption was gradually replaced by a more pluralistic orientation (Eisikovits & Beck, 1990). The need to respect parenting styles and family decision making processes came to be recognized. Only by taking parental expectations into consideration in designing residential environments could these institutions remain relevant or socially adaptive.

A discrepancy between the traditional "normalcy" ideology of residential education in Israel and the emerging needs of client populations became apparent. A great many residential settings failed to diversify their programs, and many were unable to attract quality manpower to perform increasingly complex educational tasks. Youth counselors ("Madrichim") were no longer the broadly-educated, "generalist" pioneers of the pre-statehood days (Wolins, 1971). In fact, the occupation itself dwindled into a negative or, at best, transient career choice which, in turn, contributed to the further downward spiraling of the quality of education that was offered.

Lack of communication with the outside community contributed to the isolation of the institution and to a decline in its ability to serve as an equalizer of educational opportunity. Smilansky, Kashti, and Arieli (1982) note that a considerable number of institutions they surveyed ran at high vacancy levels due to low enrollments and high dropout rates. They claimed that good community schools, offering a variety of vocational training programs, had been established in many of the development towns, traditionally housing a high concentration of new immigrant populations.

Thus, placing youth in residential schools, particularly for technical training, was no longer the only alternative. Smilansky, Kashti, and Arieli (1982) also underline the incompatibility between potential candidates in real need of placement and the willingness of institutions to accommodate them. The settings were often reluctant to admit pre-delinquent youths for fear of further compromising their waning status as normative educational options for those with academic aspirations.

The foregoing analysis leads us to conclude that residential education in Israel has reached a critical juncture. In the pre-statehood days the institution served as a cultural "maximizer" (Henry, 1965) for its charges due to the congruence between its particularistic goals and the universal values of the pioneering society. Following statehood, residential education underwent a crisis as its traditional ideology was challenged by the rapidly changing demographic picture in the larger, ethnically more heterogeneous society.

Thus, these institutions were caught between nostalgia for their glorious past and the need for radical change as a precondition for survival. By preferring the perpetuation of traditional goals and organizational structures to the introduction of substantive changes, many of them became cultural "minimizers," unable to perform their social mandate: to prepare "disadvantaged" immigrant youth to function in society. This brings us back to our initial premise. Contrary to Yehudi Cohen's skepticism about man's ability to influence the "emergence or loss" of cultural institutions, it was argued that by controlling the character of such institutions, one is actually passing a verdict on their very existence. The evolution of the Israeli residential school illustrates this.

Cohen also claims that the study of one social institution yields valuable insights into macro-social processes. What can we learn about Israeli society from this longitudinal analysis of the functions of residential education? Its impasse reflects social dilemmas regarding the equitable handling of the problems stemming from ethnic and cultural differences. Lacking the clarity of vision that characterized its earlier days, the residential school of recent times is called upon to operationalize a yet uncrystallized social philosophy.

NOTES

1. Wolins (1974) claims that this orientation is gradually changing. His research has dispelled the myth of the detrimental impact of institutional life on normal child development (Bowlby, 1952) by demonstrating that well-adjusted children live in group arrangements such as the Israeli kibbutz, the Soviet boarding school, the Austrian "kindersdorf," etc. The increasing need for out-of-home child care as a result of the dramatically rising trend of maternal employment has been another influential factor.

2. For detailed descriptions and analyses of the variety of residential educational arrangements in the pre-statehood period as well as following national independence, see Kashti, 1979; Kashti, Arieli and Wozner, 1981; and Wolins, 1981.

B. Future Potential for Normative Student Populations[1]

Thinking about the future of society actually means thinking about the future of children. Education is the most powerful vehicle for attempting to influence it. Interest in the future of any social institution one wishes to study is more than justified.

Yet the future is not a major focus in most research about residential education arrangements. Whether we talk about boarding schools for elite populations such as the British public schools, programs for new immigrant children and youth in Israel in the post-statehood period, or programs for children with behavioral or emotional difficulties such as the American residential treatment centers, residential education settings cater to populations with special needs: distinct, well defined segments of the general student

---

1. This and the following selection are adapted from R. A. Eisikovits and I. M. Schwartz, "The Future of Residential Education and Care," *Residential Treatment for Children & Youth, 8*(3), 1985, 5-19.

body. This encourages the development of a certain separatist vision on behalf of its practitioners which, in turn, reinforces the isolation of the field from the concerns of the wider educational community (Eisikovits, 1987).

As a result, neither the treatment sub-field nor boarding schools for the elite, to consider the two extremes of the spectrum, are likely to be characterized by a distinct pro-change orientation. The former regards the problems it is handling as endemic to human nature, and largely invariable. The latter are also more likely to be interested in maintaining the status quo, in which they have a somewhat privileged role, than in promoting educational change.

Nevertheless, this section examines the potential contributions of residential settings to the education of all students in the future. Most thinkers envisage education in the future to be an individual rather than mass-oriented enterprise. In the words of Shane (1981):

> Equal opportunity in education does not mean the same for everyone . . . Because of differences that exist among learners of every age, the content, methods, and organization of the curriculum should be adapted to the gradations in the level of human development. Phrased in another way, good learning is personalized learning. (p. 134)

Also stressed is the importance of incorporating beyond-the-classroom, real-life experiences into the learning process. This is believed to provide students with skills for dealing with change and to form the habit of lifelong learning.

The expectations for educational gains to accrue from these kinds of experiences are high, based on the assumption that they are meaningful enough to serve as effective catalysts for change. However, comparative studies of youth participation conducted in Israel and the U.S. (Eisikovits, Hedin, & Adam, 1982, 1984) reveal that this is seldom the case. Our findings indicate that youth are rarely involved in genuine decision- or policy-making, most seldom partake in egalitarian adult-youth interactions, and they do not usually receive the training and skills in communication, negotiation, and persuasion necessary to act effectively.

In view of this, it is argued that setting up simulated environments for maximizing such learning opportunities might be the optimal solution. Residential settings are ideally suited for this purpose due to their holistic character, designability, and territorial boundedness, i.e., their culture-like attributes. Let us consider some such options.

Intensive career orientation programs are one example. The milieu characteristic of various health-related professions or naval careers can be simulated to allow participants a short but complete immersion in the ethos of these professional cultures, which is hard to attain in any other way. Such environments would be operated by specially trained educational personnel, using up to date equipment that is made available to learners at all times.

Space research stations and agro-botanical or environmental research labs are additional options. Through operating them, youth would gain first hand experience of the kind of responsibility and commitment necessary to succeed in these areas.

Fostering intercultural dialogue among youths and the intensive study of foreign languages are also central goals on the educational futures agenda (Bear & Slaughter, 1993; Longstreet & Shane, 1993; Pesanelli, 1993). These, too, can be effectively accomplished in such purposively designed residential environments, where young people from various countries could be brought together to participate in international peace camps, seminars on global issues, leadership training institutes for students from different racial, ethnic, or social backgrounds, and intensive foreign language programs.

Because of the complexity of educational tasks in the future, no one central institution, like the present day school, is expected to provide for all the educational needs of the young (Mead, 1970). Instead, different competencies will be acquired in different and specialized settings referred to as "learning centers" (Perelman, 1992). Aided by career counselors, students will learn to draw up individual educational plans (Wirth, 1992). This is in line with another major futurist creed, namely, that education should increase rather than decrease differences in what individuals will be able to contribute to society (Longstreet & Shane, 1993). It is assumed that respect for such differences would be simultaneously instilled to allow unimpeded communication as well as a wide definition of normative behavior (Eisikovits, 1987).

In this decentralized educational scenario for the future, the distinction currently made between "normative" student populations and those with special needs, i.e., the traditional clients of residential education, would become redundant. These environments could then be redesigned and reconfigured to serve, collectively, the needs of all students.

C.
A Heuristic Approach to Service Delivery for Traditional Residential Populations

Regardless of tolerance toward diversity and a wide definition of normative behavior, Wolins and Wozner (1982) remind us that populations with special needs for whom institutionalization remains the proper answer will not disappear. Therefore, the realistic approach is to continuously improve these settings. In the field of child and youth care, adjustments will need to be made in our thinking regarding potential clients and our ability to envisage intrinsically different types of programs. Also needed are innovative approaches to the preparation of child care personnel and alternative modes of financing residential care. The following elements are considered to be indispensable for such effective usage:

- to bring out the holistic character of these environments through conscious, conceptually based program design;
- to emphasize client choice in program assignment. Clients, meaning children in consultation with their guardians, when applicable, should also have access to professional advice throughout this process;
- to formalize client consent to cooperate with program staff as a precondition for individual change and learning;
- to provide accurate descriptive literature on a variety of programs for preliminary inspection and to enable exploratory site visits for mutual assessment;
- to spell out program goals in terms of competencies to be acquired with an estimated time range necessary for mastering them. This would aid clients in basing their decisions partly on the necessary time commitment, as well as providing objective

grounds for evaluating program effectiveness and clients' individual progress;
- to re-enact choice in longer term treatment through contract renewals. The freedom to leave the program at various predetermined stages or points in time should be upheld;
- to direct accountability for service rendered toward clients rather than other professionals or funding agencies. This would result in client empowerment and overall improvement of the quality of care.

The economic implications of such an approach would be to channel funds through individual clients. This would enable them to "shop around" for the program that best suits their needs. A beneficial competitive spirit would thus be introduced, leading to structural and systemic changes in the field.

This chapter has demonstrated the paradigm-enriching effect of the cross-domain exchange of ideas. The application of the anthropological model in child and youth care worker education and training helps to prepare professionals to face the challenges of innovative planning and modes of service delivery to a wide range of youthful client populations.

Chapter 6

"Family Culture Ethnography" as an Instrument for Cultural Sensitization of Child and Youth Care Workers

Chapter 5 considered alternative future roles for child and youth care workers in innovative service delivery contexts. This chapter focuses on how to enhance the inter-cultural effectiveness of these practitioners, whose daily engagement with their charges makes value judgment and transmission an intrinsic part of their everyday work reality. The intensity of these contacts can lead to non-reflective action. As treatment stereotypes were shown to be harmfully applied in Chapter 3, the danger of using cultural stereotypes under such stressful circumstances is also real.

Faced with youngsters on a 24-hour daily basis, workers are exposed to different lifestyles, the expressions of which might clash with norms and practices in the treatment setting. Effective handling of such situations requires cultural sensitivity. This is particularly important because workers often serve as adult role models for youths who are away from their families and homes (Maluccio, 1981, 1991). Many practitioners also have direct communication with their clients' families.

Therefore, workers' awareness of their own preferences and biases, which can be achieved through a systematic examination of their family values and traditions, can enhance their successful

[Haworth co-indexing entry note]: " 'Family Culture Ethnography' as an Instrument for Cultural Sensitization of Child and Youth Care Workers" Eisikovits, Rivka A. Co-published simultaneously in *Child & Youth Services* (The Haworth Press, Inc.) Vol. 18, No. 1, 1997, pp. 79-86; and: *The Anthropology of Child and Youth Care Work* (Rivka A. Eisikovits) The Haworth Press, Inc., 1997, pp. 79-86. Single or multiple copies of this article are available from The Haworth Document Delivery Service [1-800-342-9678, 9:00 a.m. - 5:00 p.m. (EST). E-mail address: getinfo@haworth.com].

treatment relations. It is for this reason that *family culture ethnography* as an instrument for cultural awareness training is presented in this chapter. It is adaptable for use in pre-service as well as in-service training contexts.

Designing and Conducting a "Family Culture Ethnography"

Along with other educational and clinical professionals, child and youth care workers are, in effect, informally "licensed" to shape their clients' or charges' values as part of their professional mandate. Yet they are not always thoroughly equipped to understand the value implications of their interventions, nor are many of them fully aware of the value orientation that molds their own worldview and underlies their actions. Systematic cultural sensitivity training should, therefore, be an important part of the professional socialization of these workers.

The conduct of in-depth anthropological inquiry into the trainees' family cultures accomplishes this goal. To this end, I have operationalized the concept of *family culture ethnography,* turning it into a combined research/treatment tool, and I have applied it in a number of advanced-level anthropology courses with students in the human service professions.

"Teachers and Their Family Cultures," an article by Ruth Landes (1976), provided the inspiration. Though she illustrates with ample quotes from her students' papers the "enormous social variety in the origins of teachers despite the teachers' usual middle class appearance and professional oneness" (p. 401), she does not supply any detail about the mechanics of her students' projects. Thus, the reader is unaware of either the scope or content areas covered by their investigations. They were conducted, one is left to assume, in the tradition of open-ended ethnographic reporting.

Their overall intent, to sensitize teachers to their own cultural heritage to make them more effective in working with minority students–though implicit in Landes' (1976) commentary–is never directly taken up by any of the "teacher-ethnographers" (my term). She uses the expression "family culture" broadly, as coterminous with the teachers' ethnic heritage.

As I have argued in Chapter 1, families can be regarded as cultural entities according to a cognitive definition of culture. Members of a family system, nuclear or extended, command exclusive knowledge, have a specific structure, and use idiosyncratic symbolism to communicate with each other. Thus, as the basic social unit in all human communities, families function simultaneously as "carriers" of a common ethnic or national culture and as its unique expression.

It is posited that the systematic ethnographic study of practitioners' family cultures, following the above conceptualization, promotes intercultural sensitivity while maintaining a balanced stance between the nomothetic (or norm-referenced) and idiographic (or particularistic) dimensions of cultural existence. It fosters a careful examination of the value base that shapes their worldview and their actions. The instrument described herein has workers assume the role of ethnographers. In this role they are asked to explicitly address the projected implications of their ethnographic inquiry for their future professional functioning on several levels. A detailed outline is provided to facilitate systematic research. The scope and foci of the investigation can be adjusted according to individual needs and time constraints.

THE INSTRUMENT

Workers can start out by constructing a three-generational genealogical diagram of their families with the generation of their grandparents considered as number one and that of the ethnographer as number three. The information provided for all persons, in addition to their relation to the ethnographer, should include year and place of birth (and death), date of significant geographical moves or cross-cultural migration, occupation before and after the move and other relevant facts, easy to chart and visualize on a diagram, such as divorce, remarriage, adoption, etc. A legend or code for various entries may prove useful.

An introductory section should be included to describe data collection sources and methods and explain specific methodological difficulties encountered. The methods that may be employed include participant observation, interviewing, and the collection of life histories as well as the analysis of various written documents such as contracts, wills, diaries, the interpretation of family photographs, etc. In addition, an abbreviated and modified version of Kluckhohn and Strodtbeck's (1961) values test is administered to all informants. For deceased or missing informants, other family members can be requested to fill out the values test in accordance with their perception of that person's value profile. The methodological hazards of this procedure should be discussed and data obtained in this way should be interpreted with due caution. The process of collecting such data has been found to be of self-instructive value to the ethnographers, methodological inaccuracies notwithstanding (see Part III).

I have used the following instructions to guide my students in organizing their materials:

> In part I, entitled "The Family as a Cultural Unit," the first task the ethnographer has to accomplish is to establish the boundaries of this cultural unit over space and time. Students are asked to:
>
> a. trace the origin of the family from generation #1 to generation #3 in parallel manner for the maternal and paternal branches;
> b. document, analyze, and compare cross-generationally various members' views of the influences of cultural and geographical changes on the family as a unit; and
> c. examine representatives' perceptions of the role played by the family (for its individual members) throughout these processes in different generations.

While Part I considers the interplay between the family unit as a major shield and adaptive mechanism and larger outside forces, Part II concentrates on the intra-family scene. Here, students:

a. describe and compare role division patterns cross-generationally;
b. portray and analyze daily life routine through time with special reference to differences in interaction patterns among members on weekdays and on holidays;
c. describe and compare styles of celebration of a particular holiday and a specific family event;

d. analyze a crisis situation, cross-generationally where possible; the degree to which an event is seen as a crisis by one generation as compared to the others is also addressed; and
e. undertake a longitudinal study of gender-related educational aspirations, i.e., attitudes toward the education of boys and girls or boys versus girls.

In Part III, the three-generational set of results for items on the values test are presented diagrammatically and analyzed. The comparative interpretation allows for the emergence of a family's problem solving styles or patterns in a variety of life contexts. This concluding part focuses on the following three questions:

1. What did the ethnographer learn about himself or herself from the factual findings of the inquiry?
2. What did he or she learn about self from the research process?
3. In what ways can both content and process learning be utilized to improve the learner's future professional effectiveness as a child and youth care worker?

REPORTED PROCESS LEARNING ACCOMPLISHED

As the scope of this paper is limited to the presentation of *family culture ethnography* as an instrument for cultural sensitivity training, no systematic analysis of content learning elicited by various student ethnographies is undertaken. Process learning, mainly of the reflexive type, is selectively illustrated; content findings are used only for purposes of contextualization. Implications on both the personal and professional levels are included because they are considered to be codeterminant.

Several students claimed the process brought them closer to their families, as the interviews evolved into intimate discussions. Bringing up memories of shared experiences helped stress family unity. Some students specifically mentioned the positive influence these sessions had on their relationships with grandparents, who cherished the opportunity to pass on their views and stories to the ethnographer, enjoying the center-stage position the occasion offered them.

Ethnographers realized and vividly illustrated how deeply they had been affected by their family cultures. This was contradictory to the view held by many prior to the inquiry, according to which they felt that they had broken away from family traditions. The comparative analysis of their multi-generational investigation has demonstrated just how slowly values, norms, and family traditions change–an insight clearly applicable in professional encounters with clients.

The fact that so many report having been surprised by "new" information on their family history and culture indicates a general ignorance concerning things pertinent to the innermost circle of intimates. Due to this research, a historical perspective was recognized as valuable for the students' present functioning. This was often accompanied by feelings of nostalgia for information irretrievably lost. In an era of rapid change, it is easy to lose interest in the stories of one's elders as part of the individuation process. However, the reassessment of the importance of family cultural knowledge became a measure of the student ethnographers' development as reflective individuals and as professionals, bringing a realization that the two are inseparable.

Another benefit cited was the ability to see parents' and grandparents' lives and attitudes from a distance through the anthropological lenses used in this inquiry. This often had a cathartic effect, resolving long-harbored resentments from the past.

Students also pointed out the advantage accruing to their own families of procreation from being encouraged to discuss family patterns with their spouses. This yielded a better understanding of their family dynamics and enabled a more informed process of shaping its future directions.

The ethnographic research clearly demonstrated the irrelevance of ethnic family stereotypes. Thus, a heightened awareness of the importance of understanding various family styles of interaction and decision making in ethnically diverse social contexts was further dramatized. Instead, all of the student ethnographers emphasized the need to see each individual family as a potentially effective and unique coping unit with the goal of capitalizing upon its inherent strengths. Consequently, several reported having resolved to apply an abbreviated or adapted version of the *family culture ethnography* method as a routine working tool with clients.

Family culture ethnographies served as diagnostic tools in revealing to the student ethnographers certain traits in their family histories that they now came to perceive as either assets or handicaps in dealing with specific types of client problems or populations. For example, some quoted the fact of having had a cross-generational history of intact families with a militantly anti-divorce bias as an issue to be aware of when working with children from broken families and their divorced or separated parents. Others mentioned their own distinct family style of self-reliance in handling crisis situations as something to take into account in future professional encounters with families who have collateral patterns (i.e., rely on members of the extended family) or those who appeal for professional assistance. Fundamentally discrepant attitudes toward asserting parental authority between the student's family culture and that of his or her clients was also expressed as a concern.

As these inquiries were conducted in Israel, several students whose families were almost completely wiped out by the Nazi Holocaust became painfully alerted to the deficiency in sources of information regarding their family histories. Some were unable to complete the assignment and had to be referred to written historical sources as an alternative. A few exhibited hostility toward the very idea of doing a *family culture ethnography.* Other students, however, took the opposite approach and used the opportunity of having to fulfill a formal course requirement to break a family taboo, a "conspiracy of silence" as one called it, and bring this painful subject out into the open. These students reported that not only have they benefited from this, but their parents and other family members have as well.

Another gain came from having experienced the hardship of self and family probing and revelation. Ethnographers became highly sensitized to the potential hurt to family members and themselves from such exposure and devised various methods to minimize it. This, all claimed, is a hard-earned skill that will directly serve their clients. Yet at the same time, the successful completion of the research task served to boost the moral justification to direct, advise, probe, or otherwise intervene in clients' lives. The ability to alternate between the child and youth care worker's and the ethnographic researcher's roles yielded a sense of increased professional competence and dramatized how the two perspectives complement each other.

CONCLUSION

Although educated to function according to universalistic canons of knowledge, these future practitioners are also cultural beings. So are their clients, with whom they engage in mutual interpretations of acts and actions colored by their respective cultural identities. *Family culture ethnography* as an instrument for cultural sensitivity training demonstrates one possible contribution of the anthropological approach to the socialization of students for professional careers in child and youth care work.

Concluding Remarks

The potential uses of an anthropological model of child and youth care work have been examined in this volume. With its emphasis on context, on the subjective construction of meaning, and on the interplay among multiple identities due to participants' simultaneous membership in several culture-bearing units, this approach can enhance workers' on-the-job effectiveness with clients and co-workers and improve intra- and inter-organizational communication with other human service professionals.

The model offers an organic continuum between everyday work experience and conceptual practice, organizing seemingly haphazard events into a systematized body of knowledge. Although providing specific skills, it is more than a technology; it is a humanistic worldview from which a humanistic practice philosophy can be derived.

The broadening of horizons provided by the cultural perspective equips child and youth care workers to transcend narrowly drawn, task-specific role definitions and organizational boundaries and helps them perform successfully in a rapidly changing social context that requires constant assessment of needs and evaluation of performance. In other words, it prepares child and youth care workers to face the challenges of a dynamic, emergent profession.

[Haworth co-indexing entry note]: "Concluding Remarks." Eisikovits, Rivka A. Co-published simultaneously in *Child & Youth Services* (The Haworth Press, Inc.) Vol. 18, No. 1, 1997, p. 87; and: *The Anthropology of Child and Youth Care Work* (Rivka A. Eisikovits) The Haworth Press, Inc., 1997, p. 87. Single or multiple copies of this article are available from The Haworth Document Delivery Service [1-800-342-9678, 9:00 a.m. - 5:00 p.m. (EST). E-mail address: getinfo@haworth.com].

References

Alcoholics Anonymous World Service, Inc. (1952). *Twelve steps and twelve traditions*. New York: AA World Service, Inc.

Argyris, C., Putnam, R., & Smith, D.M. (1985). *Action Science*. San Francisco: Jossey-Bass Publishers.

Argyris, C., & Shon, D. (1974). *Theory in practice: Increasing professional effectiveness*. San Francisco: Jossey-Bass Publishers.

Aronowitz, S., & Giroux, H. (1993). *Education still under siege*. Westport, CT: Bergin & Garvey.

Atkinson, P. (1992). *Understanding ethnographic texts*. Newbury Park, CA: Sage.

Bear, M., & Slaughter, R. (1993). *Education for the twenty-first century*. London: Routledge.

Beker, J. (1989). On the nature of modifying environments. *Child and Youth Care Quarterly, 18*(3), 159-160.

Beker, J., & Baizerman, M. (1982). Professionalization in child and youth care and the context of the work: Some new perspectives. *Journal of Child Care, 1*(1), 11-20.

Beker, J., & Barnes, H. (1990). The educateur returns to America: Approaching the development of professional child and youth care cross-culturally through ILEX. *Child and Youth Care Quarterly, 19* (3), 161-175.

Bellah, R., Madsen, R., Sullivan, W., Swidler, A., & Tipton, S. (1985). *Habits of the heart: Individualism and commitment in American life*. New York: Harper & Row.

Bowlby, J. (1952). *Maternal care and mental health* (2nd Ed.). Geneva: World Health Organization.

Bronfenbrenner, U. (1970). *Two worlds of childhood: U.S. and U.S.S.R.* New York: Russell Sage Foundation.

Burnett, J. (1973). Event description and analysis in the microethnography of urban classrooms. In F. Ianni & E. Storey (Eds.), *Cultural relevance and educational issues*. Boston: Little, Brown and Co.

Clifford, J. (1986). On ethnographic authority. In J. Clifford (Ed.), *The predicament of culture* (pp. 21-54). Cambridge, MA: Harvard University Press.

Cohen, Y.A. (1975). The state system, schooling, and cognitive and motivational patterns. In N.K. Shimahara & A. Scrupski (Eds.), *Social forces and schooling: An anthropological and sociological perspective* (pp. 6-36). New York: David McKay Company, Inc.

de Chardin, T. (1965). *The Phenomenon of Man*. New York: Harper & Row.

Dobbert, M.L. (1975). Another route to a general theory of culture transmission: A systems model. *Anthropology and Education Quarterly, 6,* 22-26.

Dobbert, M.L. (1982). *Ethnographic research: Theory and application for modern schools and societies*. New York: Praeger.

Dobbert, M.L., & Eisikovits, R.A. (1984). *Observing learning in everyday settings: A guide to the holistic study of cultural transmission/acquisition in daily life*. Minneapolis: University of Minnesota, mimeo.

Dobbert, M.L., & Kurth-Shai, R. (1992). Systematic ethnography: Toward an evolutionary science of education and culture. In M.D. LeCompte, W.L. Milroy, & J. Preissle (Eds.), *Handbook of qualitative research in education* (pp. 93-159). San Diego, CA: Academic Press.

Durkin, R. (1990). Competency, relevance, and empowerment: A case for restructuring of children's programs. *Child & Youth Services, 13*(1), 105-117.

Eisenstadt, S.N. (1973). *Israeli society.* London: Weidenfeld and Nicolson.

Eisikovits, R.A. (1980). The cultural scene of a juvenile treatment center for girls: Another look. *Child Care Quarterly, 9*(3), 158-174.

Eisikovits, R.A. (1983). No exit: Residential treatment and the "sick role" trap. *Child Care Quarterly, 12*(1), 36-44.

Eisikovits, R.A. (1985). Children's institutions in Israel as mirrors of social and cultural change. *Child & Youth Services, 7*(3/4), 21-28.

Eisikovits, R.A. (1987). Roles for residential settings in the education of tomorrow's youth. In Y. Kashti & M. Arieli (Eds.), *Resi-*

dential settings and the community: Congruence and conflict (pp. 301-313). London: Freund.

Eisikovits, R.A. (1991). The child care worker as ethnographer: Uses of the anthropological approach in residential child and youth care worker education and practice. In J. Beker & Z. Eisikovits (Eds.), *Knowledge utilization in residential child and youth care practice* (pp. 275-290). Washington, DC: Child Welfare League of America.

Eisikovits, R.A., & Beck, R. (1990). Models governing the education of new immigrant children in Israel. *Comparative Education Review, 34*(2), 177-195.

Eisikovits, R.A., & Eisikovits, Z. (1980). Detotalizing the institutional experience: The role of the school in the residential treatment of juveniles. *Residential and Community Child Care Administration, 1*(4), 365-373.

Eisikovits, R.A., Hedin, D.P., & Adam, V. (1982). Models of effective youth organization: A comparative study. *New Designs for Youth Development,* Nov/Dec., 9-19.

Eisikovits, R.A., Hedin, D.P., & Adam, V. (1984). Political participation: A comparative view of Israeli and American youth. *Children and Youth Services Review, 6*(1), 47-64.

Eisikovits, R.A., & Schwartz, I.M. (1991). The future of residential education and care. *Residential Treatment for Children & Youth, 8*(3), 5-19.

Eisikovits, Z., Beker, J., & Guttmann, E. (1991). The known and the used in residential child and youth care work. In J. Beker & Z. Eisikovits (Eds.), *Knowledge utilization in residential child and youth care practice* (pp. 3-23). Washington, DC: Child Welfare League of America.

Elboim-Dror, R. (1989). Conflict and consensus in educational policy making in Israel. In E. Krausz (Ed.), *Education in a comparative context* (pp. 45-52). New Brunswick, NJ: Transaction Publishers.

Ferguson, R.V. (1990). Distance education: Catch the wave. *Child & Youth Services, 13*(2), 263-274.

Ferguson, R.V. (1993). Child and youth care education: Approaching a new millenium. *Child and Youth Care Forum, 22*(4), 251-261.

Frankel, B. (1987). Comment on *Anthropology as interpretive quest,* by Roger M. Keesing. *Current Anthropology, 28*(2), 169-170.

Frankenstein, K. (1951). To the problem of ethnic differences. *Megamot, 2,* 261-276 (in Hebrew).

Frankenstein, K. (1961). The school without parents. *Megamot, 12,* 3-23 (in Hebrew).

Garduque, L., & Peters, D.L. (1982). Toward rapprochement in child care research: An optimistic view. *Child Care Quarterly, 11*(1), 12-21.

Gauthier, P. (1990).Development of a new approach to emotionally deprived children and youth. *Child & Youth Services, 13*(1), 71-79.

Gearing, F. (1974). Where we are and where we might go from here: Steps toward a general theory of cultural transmission. *Council on Anthropology and Education Newsletter, 4*(1), 1-10.

Geertz, C. (1973). *The interpretation of cultures*. New York: Basic Books.

Geertz, C. (1988). *Works and lives*. Stanford, CA: Stanford University Press.

Goffman, E. (1959). *The presentation of self in everyday life*. New York: Doubleday, Anchor.

Goffman, E. (1961). *Asylums*. New York: Doubleday, Anchor.

Goodenough, H. (1966). *Cooperation in change: An anthropological approach to community development.* New York: Science Editions, John Wiley & Sons.

Gouldner, A.W. (1975). Sociology and everyday life. In L.T. Coser (Ed.), *The idea of social structure: Papers in honor of Robert K. Merton*. New York: Harcourt Brace.

Grupper, E., & Eisikovits, R. (1993). Fostering moratorium in residential child and youth care education. *Child and Youth Care Forum, 22*(3), 177-192.

Guttmann, E. (1991). Immediacy in residential child and youth care: The fusion of experience, self-consciousness, and action. In J. Beker & Z. Eisikovits (Eds.), *Knowledge utilization in residential child and youth care practice* (pp. 65-82). Washington, DC: Child Welfare League of America.

Hansen, J.F. (1979). *Sociocultural perspectives on human learning:*

An introduction to educational anthropology. Englewood Cliffs, NJ: Prentice Hall.

Henry, J. (1960). Cross cultural outline of education. *Current Anthropology, 1,* 267-305.

Henry, J. (1965). *Culture against man*. New York: Random House.

Jones, H.D. (1985). The profession at work in contemporary society. In H.D. Jones, M. Courtioux, J. Kalcher, W. Tuggener, & K. Waaldijk (Eds.), *The social pedagogue in Europe: Living with others as a profession* (pp. 74-108). Zurich: FICE International.

Kaplan, D., & Manners, R. (1972). *Culture theory*. Englewood Cliffs, NJ: Prentice Hall.

Kashti, Y. (1979). *The socializing community: Disadvantaged adolescents in Israeli youth villages*. Ramat Aviv, Israel: School of Education, Tel Aviv University.

Kashti, Y. (1993). *Boarding schools and changes in society and culture.* Tel Aviv, Israel: Ramot Press (in Hebrew).

Kashti, Y, Arieli, M., & Wozner, Y. (1981). *The Israeli residential setting: Tradition, social context, organization* (Report of the Israeli-American seminar on out-of-school education, Residential education in Israel). Jerusalem: The Ministry of Education and Culture.

Kerlinger, F.N. (1989). *Foundations of behavioral research* (3rd ed.). New York: Holt, Rinehart & Winston.

Kluckhohn, F., & Strodtbeck, F. (1961). *Variations in value orientations*. Evanston, IL: Peterson.

Kroeber, A.L., & Kluckhohn, C. (1952). Culture: A critical review of concepts and definitions. *Harvard University Papers of the Peabody Museum of American Archaeology and Ethnology,* #47.

Landes, R. (1976). Teachers and their family cultures. Reprinted in J. Roberts & J. Akinsanya (Eds.), *Schooling in the cultural context* (pp. 401-420). New York: McKay Co.

LeCompte, M.D., & Preissle, J., with Tesch, R. (1993). *Ethnography and qualitative design in educational research* (2nd ed.). Orlando, FL: Academic Press.

Levine, S., & Kozloff, M. (1978). The sick-role: Assessment and overview. *Annual Review of Sociology, 4,* 317-343.

Longstreet, W., & Shane, H. (1993). *Curriculum for a new millennium*. Boston: Allyn & Bacon.

Maier, H.W. (1990). A developmental perspective for child and youth care work. *Child & Youth Services,* 13(1), 25-40.
Maier, H.W. (1991). Developmental foundations of child and youth care work. In J. Beker & Z. Eisikovits (Eds.), *Knowledge utilization in residential child and youth care practice* (pp. 25-48). Washington, DC: Child Welfare League of America.
Maluccio, A.N. (1981). Promoting client and worker competence in child welfare. In *The Social Welfare Forum–1980* (pp. 136-153). New York: Columbia University Press.
Maluccio, A.N. (1991). Interpersonal and group life in residential care: A competence-centered, ecological perspective. In J. Beker & Z. Eisikovits (Eds.), *Knowledge utilization in residential child and youth care practice* (pp. 49-63). Washington, DC: Child Welfare League of America.
Mead, M. (1970). *Culture and commitment: The study of the generation gap*. Garden City, NY: Doubleday.
Newman, L.W. (1994). *Social research methods: Quantitative and qualitative approaches*. Boston: Allyn & Bacon.
Ogbu, J. (1987). Variability in minority school performance: A problem in search of an explanation. *Anthropology and Education Quarterly, 18*(4), 312-334.
Paget, M.A. (1990). Performing the text. *Journal of Contemporary Ethnography, 19*(1), 136-155.
Parsons, T. (1957). The social system. New York: Free Press.
Pearson, L. (1990). *Children of Glasnost: Growing up Soviet.* Seattle: University of Washington Press.
Pelto, P., & Pelto, G. (1978). *Anthropological research: The structure of inquiry.* New York: Praeger.
Pence, A.R. (1990). Worlds apart? Integrating research and practice in professional child and youth care training. *Child & Youth Services, 13*(2), 235-241.
Perelman, L. (1992). *School's out: Hyperlearning, the new technology, and the end of education.* New York: Morrow.
Pesanelli, D. (1993). The plug-in school: A learning environment for the 21st century. *The Futurist,* Sept.-Oct., 29-32.
Phelan, J. (1990). Child care supervision: The neglected skill. *Child & Youth Services, 13*(1), 131-141.
Pitman, M.A., Eisikovits, R.A., & Dobbert, M.L. (1989). *Culture*

acquisition: A holistic approach to human learning. New York: Praeger.

Puttkamer, J.V. (1983). The future: Do we have a choice? *Educational Leadership, 41*(1), 4-8.

Reiter, S., & Bryen, D.N. (1991). Promoting social competence: Implications of work with mentally retarded children and adults in residential settings. In J. Beker & Z. Eisikovits (Eds.), *Knowledge utilization in residential child and youth care practice* (pp. 99-122). Washington, DC: Child Welfare League of America.

Rose, D. (1990). *Living the ethnographic life*. Newbury Park, CA: Sage.

Rottenschtreich, N. (1951). Absolute measures. *Megamot, 2,* 327-338 (in Hebrew).

Sanjek, R. (Ed.). (1990). *Fieldnotes: The making of anthropology*. Ithaca, NY: Cornell University Press.

Sanjek, R. (1991). The ethnographic present. *Man: The Journal of the Royal Anthropological Institute, 26*(4), 609-628.

Savicki, V. (1993). Clarification of child and youth care identity through an analysis of work environment and burnout. *Child and Youth Care Forum, 22*(6), 441-457.

Schon, D.A. (1987). *Educating the reflective practitioner.* San Francisco: Jossey-Bass.

Schon, D.A. (Ed.). (1991). *The reflective turn: Case studies in and on educational practice*. New York: Teachers College Press.

Seidl, F. (1974). Community-oriented residental care: The state of the art. *Child Care Quarterly, 3*(1), 150-163.

Shane, H., & Tabler, B. (1981). *Educating for a new millennium.* Bloomington, IN: The Phi Delta Kappa Educational Foundation.

Smilansky, M., Kashti, Y., & Arieli, M. (1982). *The residential education alternative*. Haifa: Ach Publishing House.

Spindler, G.D. (1975). From omnibus to linkages: Cultural transmission models. *Council on Anthropology and Education Newsletter, 5.*

Spindler, G.D. (1987). Roots revisited: Three decades of perspectives. In G.D.Spindler (Ed.), *Education and cultural process* (2nd edition, pp. 70-77). Prospect Heights, IL: Waveland.

Spindler, G.D., & Spindler, L. (1982). Roger Harker and Schonhausen: From the familiar to the strange and back again. In G.D.

Spindler (Ed.), *Doing the ethnography of schooling* (pp. 20-46). New York: Holt Rinehart.

Spindler, G.D., & Spindler, L., with Trueba, H., & Williams, M. (1990). *The American cultural dialogue and its transmission*. London: Falmer Press.

Spradley, J.P. (Ed.). (1972). *Culture and cognition*. New York: Chandler.

Spradley, J.P. (1980). *Participant observation*. New York: Holt, Rinehart & Winston.

VanderVen, K. (1993). Advancing child and youth care: A model for integrating theory and practice through connecting education, training, and the service system. *Child and Youth Care Forum, 22*(4), 263-284.

Vogt, L., Jordan, K., & Tharp, R. (1987). Explaining school failure, producing school success: Two cases. *Anthropology and Education Quarterly, 18*(4), 276-286.

Vorrath, H., & Brendtro, L. (1974). *Positive Peer culture*. Chicago: Aldine Publishing Co.

Wallace, A.F.C. (1961). Schools in revolutionary and conservative societies. In F.C. Gruber (Ed.), *Anthropology and education*. Philadelphia: University of Pennsylvania Press.

Werner, O., & Schoepfle, G.M. (1987). *Systematic fieldwork: Vol. 1, Foundations of ethnography and interviewing*. Newbury Park, CA: Sage.

Werner, O., & Schoepfle, G.M. (1987). *Systematic fieldwork: Vol. 2, Ethnographic analysis and data management*. Newbury Park, CA: Sage.

Whiting, J. (1968). *Field guide for a study of socialization*. New York: Wiley.

Whittaker, J. (1979). *Caring for troubled children*. San Francisco: Jossey-Bass Publishers.

Wilcox, K. (1982). Differential socialization in the classroom: Implications for equal opportunity. In G.D. Spindler (Ed.), *Doing the ethnography of schooling* (pp. 268-309). New York: Holt, Rinehart and Winston.

Wirth, A. (1992). *Education and work for the year 2000: Choices we face*. San Francisco: Jossey-Bass Publishers.

Wolcott, H. F. (1982). The anthropology of learning. *Anthropology and Education Quarterly, 13*(2), 83-108.

Wolcott, H .F. (1982). Mirrors, models, and monitors: Educator adaptation of the ethnographic innovation. In G.D. Spindler (Ed.), *Doing the ethnography of schooling* (pp. 68-95). New York: Holt, Rinehart and Winston.

Wolcott, M.F. (1990). *Writing up qualitative research*. Newbury Park, CA: Sage.

Wolcott, M.F. (1994). *Transforming qualitative data*. Thousand Oaks, CA: Sage.

Wolins, M. (1971). Youth Aliyah: Cause and function. In M. Wolins & M. Gottesmann (Eds.), *Group care: An Israeli approach* (pp. 3-26). New York: Gordon & Breach.

Wolins, M. (Ed.). (1974). *Successful group care: Explorations in the powerful environment*. Chicago: Aldine.

Wolins M., & Wozner, Y. (1982). *Revitalizing residential settings*. San Francisco, CA: Jossey-Bass Publishers.

Wozner, Y. (1991). *People care in institutions: A conceptual schema and its application*. New York: The Haworth Press, Inc. (Also published as *Child & Youth Services, 15*(1).)